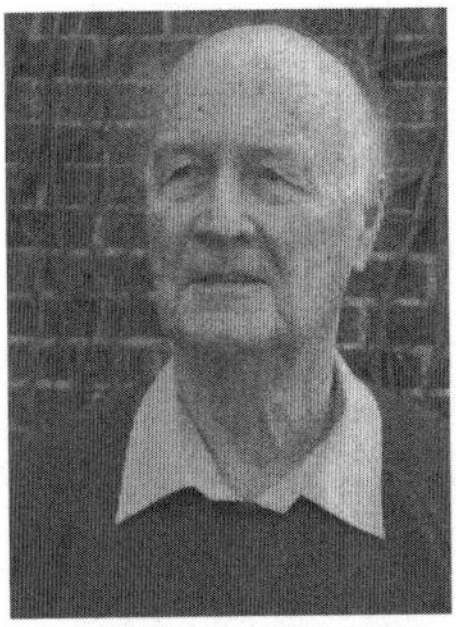

MICHAEL SPENCE was born in 1931 in Kenya. When he was 15, his family returned to England where he attended Michael Hall School. After graduation and national service in the army, he worked variously in a London shipping office, for the Kenya Police and in a finance company. At the age of 36 he was invited by Francis Edmunds to join a group of people developing Emerson College. Michael was closely involved in its evolution, carrying responsibilities for finances, administration and the campus. He also ran study groups and lectured on the threefold nature of social life at Emerson College, North America and elsewhere, and is the author of *Freeing the Human Spirit* (1999) and *After Capitalism* (2012).

THE STORY OF EMERSON COLLEGE

Its Founding Impulse, Work and Form

MICHAEL SPENCE

TEMPLE LODGE

Temple Lodge Publishing
Hillside House, The Square
Forest Row, RH18 5ES

www.templelodge.com

Published by Temple Lodge 2013

A catalogue record for this book is available from the British Library

ISBN 978 1 906999 44 5

Cover by
Typeset by DP Photosetting, Neath, West Glamorgan
Printed and bound by Berforts Ltd., Herts.

Contents

Introduction

My wife, Roswitha, and I joined Emerson College in March 1967, in the middle of its fifth year. The college as it was then and in the following years no longer exists today.

'Has anything been written of its history?' is a question that has often been asked when the early days of the college have been talked about. The answer has always been 'No, but I hope one day someone will write it.' It seemed to me that there was much in the story of Emerson that was important and that would be of interest not only to people who had been connected to the college as students, staff or supporters, but to anyone working in or hoping to start such an impulse, or in the question as to how to bring anthroposophy into actual practice in our institutions.

It never occurred to me that I could or should write something myself; I felt I did not have the talents to do such an important task justice. But there came a time when it suddenly struck me—if I did not do so, who would? There was no one else still alive who had been so actively and centrally involved as myself ever since 1967—the middle of the final year in the 'Huts'. In the following 20 to 25 years I had been a member of all the main decision-making meetings and my work took me into all non-teaching areas of the college, as well as some teaching activities. I also gave morning course lectures and ran study groups in the Foundation Year and sometimes also in the Agriculture and the Education Courses. I was now better placed than anyone else to access and use what records still existed of the founding and early years in Clent. So it seemed to me I had a certain responsibility to do what I could; I felt 'The Story of Emerson' had to be written.

But I did feel a certain inadequacy. This would be something very different from anything I had written before, a sort of biography. It seemed to me it would need very different skills from any I had ever needed. I was already 79 years old. I had never found writing easy and now felt my creative powers already considerably weaker than earlier. Despite my deteriorating memory and the lack of sufficient records, I did feel I could write a reasonable history of the college giving details of its founding, its structure, and growth and giving basic facts about the courses offered and the numbers of students and staff. But that was not what was important. What was important was to give some idea of how it came to be such a special place in so many people's lives.

So many students after leaving have spoken of what a special place it was, of how it changed their lives, how they found here something that gave them a new sense of purpose and direction. Emerson was a special place, different from anywhere else they had previously experienced. The word 'special' has constantly been used in descriptions of Emerson. Many whom I met again on my travels in later years, or when they came back for a visit, spoke of their time at Emerson 30 or even 40 years earlier as being the most important time of their lives, a time that changed them profoundly, and so often it has been the way they have said this that has added emphasis to their statement. Others who have not themselves been to the college but have met or worked with people who have done so, have asked what it is about the college that has led former students to speak so highly of it and as such a special place.

But it was not only students who saw something different or special about Emerson. I increasingly became aware that many people coming to the college in various capacities, such as contractors, consultants, inspectors, trades people, and accountants would at some time ask a question such as 'What is this place—it is different?' These were mostly people who had no connection with anthroposophy or interest in any spiritual movement—people from the world at large whose work brought them briefly to the college. But they saw or sensed something

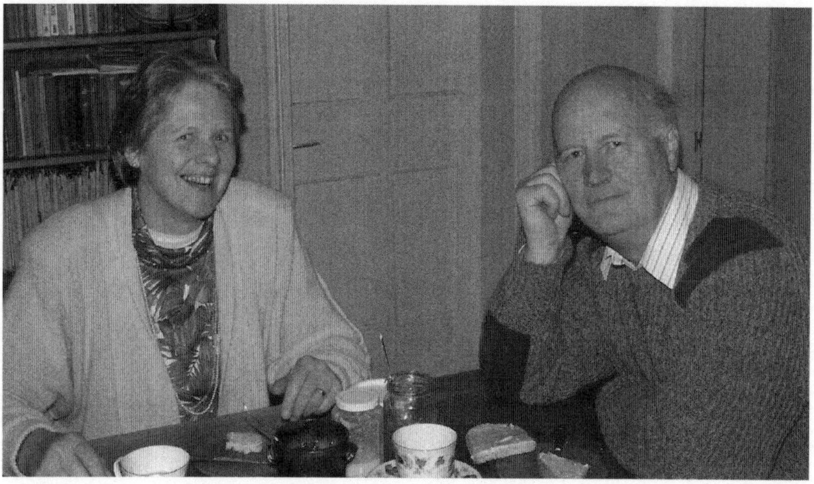

Roswitha and Michael Spence

different at Emerson. As I tried to observe this carefully it became increasingly clear to me that far more people than we realize, or who themselves recognize, do in fact become aware of things that are not perceptible to their ordinary senses. The question that I carried for a long time was 'What did they see that prompted the question in them?'

What was it about Emerson College that played such an important part in the lives of so many young people? That, to me, seemed to be the crucial question that needed to be answered in any book about the college. Could I give a reasonable and true answer to that question? I could but try. I feel certain that it was due, in good measure, to the fact that through anthroposophy, not only the teaching but the social fabric and the whole administrative and financial structure of the college was informed by a knowledge of, and commitment to, the Worlds of Spirit and to humanity in this age of the awakening Consciousness Soul. Although I felt I had some understanding of this I was not so confident that I could explain it in such a book.

The story of Emerson would not be a true picture without descriptions of the very many people who made it what it was. For me this presented a very real problem, one that lay deeply behind my feeling of inadequacy. I myself have always found it almost impossible to put into words, to paint a word picture, of individual people, their individual character and qualities of soul, their questions, life impulses, and the nature of the wisdom each brings to his or her studies or work and everything that makes each of us unique. Any book about Emerson would need to include much about the people, not just about Francis and Elizabeth Edmunds, John Davy and a few others, but about all the people who gave it form and life, whether as students, teachers, cooks, gardeners, accountants, administrators or in the many other activities. Emerson was really a working together, a sum total of all the life's paths, the working of karma and the fulfilling of pre-birth impulses and intentions of so many people, both staff and students. Every person who came to Emerson in some way touched it and changed it. Each year had its own biography. It was never an institution to which people came and passed through without leaving any mark on it.

So this is not just a history of Emerson College. It is my attempt to write my recollections of people and events, but more particularly of the anthroposophical spiritual basis that formed the bedrock on which the college was built. I do believe that, amongst other things, it was the recognition of the reality of the spirit that informed all aspects of the college life and organization that made it such a unique place to which so many people, mostly young but also older, came. Did they find at Emerson an expression of something which, in their descent from spiritual worlds into this life between birth and death, they had already sensed of the social and spiritual life of humanity that was striving to come into being?

I decided that I would take the story of Emerson into the 1980s, to the deaths of John Davy in 1984 and Francis Edmunds in 1989. That was the period when, it seems to me, the college was in the fullness of its growth and its task. It was then that a decline in student numbers began. This was not just because John and Francis died. Applications for the Foundation Year showed the first signs of falling off for the year starting September 1981, following which there was a continuing but slow and fluctuating decline. The college also changed in many other ways. I also knew that to give a true account of what happened and why during those following years would be beyond my capacity.

The book is also, as far as I have been able to make it, a record of approximately the first 25 years of the college, of the people who, in the main, formed and carried its life and work and of the courses offered. It is also a record of the forming of the inner structure of the spiritual and social guiding and decision-making processes and of the growth and development of the outer physical body of the college. I was not involved in the first four and a half years of its life, so for this I have had to depend on what I was told by Francis Edmunds himself and by others, and also from documents such as the progress reports that Francis regularly wrote to his supporters and friends.

I have also had the pleasure of talking to and hearing from many people who were here as students or staff at sometime during those early years. This has been an enormous help in reminding me, not only of people and events but also of the evolving life and activities experienced, of difficulties overcome, and important personal meetings that changed people's lives.

Though I have done some teaching, I have always seen myself as an administrator. I found that work enormously rewarding and I would not have changed it for anything. It kept me directly involved in all aspects of college life. I also had a fair idea of what went on in the courses from the meetings and from talking to students.

My hope is that the reader will find what I have written as interesting and satisfying as I have in the remembering, researching, and writing of it. My apologies for any errors, of which I am sure there must be more than I would like, and for omissions of which inevitably there are many. Another person, for example one of the teachers, writing such a story of Emerson would, no doubt, paint a very different picture from that which I give here. But it would not necessarily be less true. I was an administrator, so I see it, and cannot really do other than write of it, from that perspective. Of necessity, much of the deep concerns and deliberations that went into the planning and teaching of the courses are not included here.

But I do believe that what made Emerson College such a special experience for so many people was to be found particularly in the Foundation Year, but also in so many aspects of the life of the college as a whole. It is of this that I have attempted to write.

1
The Need for Emerson College

In the '60s and '70s of the last century, amongst those born towards the end of the Second World War and during the years immediately following, there were many in whom deep questions arose. They found expression in such movements as the Hippies and the student upheavals in universities. Many rejected the rigidities and values of the society into which they had been born, they rebelled against old hierarchical structures and codes of behaviour and a morality based on the blood, family, religion, and nationality, and against a society dominated by an economic life in which egoism flourished. They did not want to belong to any particular group, but to be free to be individual, to be themselves.

This was a time when in certain representative parts of humanity the dawning of the consciousness soul took an important step forward. The individual demanded to be recognized primarily as an individual human being, rather than as a member of a group. This awakening to consciousness of self as an individual and unique human being led to a recognition on the one side of individual human rights and, on the other, of one all-world-humanity. The anti-apartheid movement which swept through large parts of the world came out of this and was an important expression of it, as was the anti-segregation movement in America and the widespread adoption of human rights legislation by an increasing number of countries.

It came as something new in human evolution. For the first time people began to recognize in each individual human being something that was universal or 'all-human'. So the concept of individual human rights applying to all people equally came slowly to be recognized in ever wider circles. In almost all countries it has now become established in law. But it also met strong opposition. The roots of this evolving perception of the human being can be traced to much earlier times, but it emerged with considerable upheaval during the last century, most particularly during the '60s and '70s. It was an enormous change in human consciousness.

The further back we look into human evolution the more we will see that the individual human being was primarily a member of a group bound through the blood, a member of a family, tribe or people. He did not have a separate identity of his own but thought, felt and acted according to the ways of his people. His spirit was in large part the spirit of his people. Marriage, for example, was primarily an affair of the tribe or people for the maintenance of the bloodline. Marriage outside this group was not tolerated as it weakened the bloodline of the group, and weakened also the particular religion to which the group was bound through the blood. Something of this still lives on today.

The single person was born into a particular place in the group where he fulfilled a particular function, whether this was as a worker in the fields, a craftsman, trader, soldier or a priest. Society was hierarchical; all wisdom, direction and the social ordering of the people came from above through the mystery centres, the prophets and the leaders.

But since the Mystery of Golgotha this is all changing. When something new enters into human evolution it has first to appear in certain individuals. The first indication was given when the disciples of Christ Jesus, gathered together 10 days after the Ascension on the day of Pentecost, experienced the Holy Spirit.

As the disciples were together at Pentecost, the ancient festival of their people, waiting in expectation and deep devotion, there came first the experience of the 'rushing mighty wind'. Through this their souls were raised to a vision of what was to come in future epochs of time. Then there appeared the 'tongues of fire' which sat upon each one, and each was filled with the Holy Ghost. Rudolf Steiner tells us that this Holy Ghost as it is called in the Bible, or Holy Spirit, is that spirit which was formerly the spirit of the people but which now, individualized, descended on to each disciple individually. The disciples, looking far into future time, experienced that they would be able to proclaim spiritual truths which would be heard and understood by all peoples over all parts of the world; that ultimately all people would receive and understand the same truths. The Holy Spirit that hovered over each disciple as the tongues of fire was one that related to all humanity, that made a person feel himself a member, not of a particular tribe or people, but of humanity as a whole. So the disciples felt themselves, each in their own way, not as members of a particular people, but as individuals connected to, and able to speak to, the one humanity.

Thus at Whitsun the possibility was given first to the disciples, the first to understand the Christ gift to mankind, to raise themselves beyond all that comes from their inheritance, from their bodily nature, and from their particular people through the blood. This that at Pentecost was given to the disciples is destined to enter ever more strongly into all humanity; the possibility has been given for more and more people, out of their own purified forces, to bring to birth the free spirit within them.

In a lecture Rudolf Steiner gave in Hamburg on Whitsunday in 1910 he said:

> *In regard to our future growth therefore, this Holy Spirit is for us men the Spirit of development into free manhood, into the free human soul. The Spirit of freedom holds sway in that Spirit which poured itself out over the first people who had an understanding of Christianity in the first Christian Pentecostal festival, the Spirit whose most significant characteristic was indicated by Christ Himself: 'You shall know the truth, and the truth shall make you free!' Man can become free only in the spirit. So long as he is dependent on that bodily nature in which his spirit dwells, so long does he remain its slave. He can become free, only when he finds himself again in spirit, and from out of the spirit becomes lord over that which is in him. 'To become free' presupposes the discovery of oneself as a spirit within oneself. The true spirit in which we can make this discovery is the universal human spirit, which we recognise as the Pentecostal power of the Holy Spirit entering into us, and which we must bring to birth in ourselves and allow to come to manifestation.**

Although now, in our time, the rise of democracy and the concept of the equality of all people is beginning to change the old social forms, the hierarchical social structure is still the basic form of almost all our social institutions and organizations. From government to businesses and schools there is some form of head such as a prime minister or president, a chief executive officer or a head teacher. Wisdom, direction, authority and leadership are still seen as coming from above.

So too today, economic life and money have become dominant factors and to an increasing extent have taken over from religion and the blood connection as giving purpose and direction to human life. Instead of the family or tribe, it is now the organization or institution that has become primary and the individual too often secondary, an employee, to be hired or fired as needed. The ordinary person, in order to live, must sell something of himself, his labour, in order to have money to buy what he needs, 'to buy his bread'.

Over against this, against all that has come from the past and as direction from above, there has grown with increasing power the questions as to

* Rudolf Steiner, 'Whitsun, the Festival of the Free Individuality', in *The Festivals and their Meaning* (Rudolf Steiner Press, 2002).

where the emerging single free individualized human being stands. Can he find a place within social life where he can be himself and contribute to that society freely out of his own capacities and individuality? More and more people, especially the young of the 1960s and '70s, could no longer accept what came to them as wisdom, direction and morality from an outer authority. They sensed they had to find it from within themselves and they sought ways to do this. They looked for a new form of society, one in which every human being had an equal right to a place and in which each would be free to be himself. They stood at an important point in human evolution. What many sensed within themselves was that which for some five centuries had been in preparation and was now trying to be born—out of the group based on the blood the free separate individual had to be liberated.

In about 1965, shortly before I became involved in Emerson College, I read an article in a newspaper which gave me pause for thought. A reporter had met some hippies walking along a country road. They were a comparatively new phenomenon at that time. He asked them where they were going and they told him they were 'looking for Man'. Who or what was this man they were looking for? On the surface this was an extraordinary answer, but the reporter obviously experienced it as a very serious one, one that reflected something of what was driving the young people on their search. This man seemed to be something they were not but that they could become, but that first they had to find.

For me this reflected a question I myself had had earlier. In my late 20s, at a particular moment and place I can remember quite clearly, I had come to the question that can roughly be expressed as 'Who, or what, am I?' I had come suddenly to the realization that almost all my opinions, beliefs, moral and other values, political orientation and ideas of right and wrong, good and bad, came from the family and people into which I had been born and the place in society in which I was raised—I was a white, upper-middle class male born on a farm in Kenya in an old colonial family. But where was I myself? Where were the opinions and ideas that I myself had come to out of my own activity? Where were the beliefs and certainties that I had come to out of my own searching? It seemed to me that over 95 per cent of what I thought was me was in fact not me but an expression of something else. And the question arose within me 'How do I find or become myself?'

Later, after I had come to Emerson, there was a revealing article in *The Times* newspaper. This was at the time of the Vietnamese war. There was still conscription then in America, but many young men refused their call-up. Many went abroad to avoid it. Others ritually burnt their call-up papers. Some were sent to prison. The reporter spoke to a group of these young men from America and asked them why they refused to fight. The answer he quoted was very indicative of the time. They said that they recognized that the North Vietnamese were the aggressors, that there may well be something evil about them, 'But they are also human and who am I to go and shoot one?' It was as though in many of these young people there was a dawning recognition that in the other human being, whoever he may be, even him with whom outwardly he had nothing in common, with whom there might be serious disagreement, and even enmity, there was also that of the nature of the Divine which he sensed, however dimly, in the depths of his own soul. In this was dawning the recognition of the single free and independent human being within one humanity.

Francis Edmunds understood, or sensed, something of the evolutionary forces working in humanity, and he felt connected to, and had an understanding for, what lived and strove in the young people, particularly in America of the counterculture and the hippy generation. He saw it as a spiritual awakening, but one confused and hindered by the education, materialism, and growing technology. But amongst all these young people there were some who had come through birth bringing with them strong intentions to find a path to the Spirit and from the Spirit to bring healing forces to human society and the Earth. It was for these that Francis Edmunds founded Emerson College.

Francis himself as a younger man had had similar questions. He understood something of what this later generation was looking for and saw clearly that only the anthroposophical path of inner development could lead to the answers for which they were looking. They had brought their questions with them through birth from spiritual worlds from which they had come. Out of their own pre-birth resolves they had first to awaken within themselves the consciousness soul. For this they needed a place where they could meet the active spirit in practice and where they could find the path to their work in the world. But it was not a question of just teaching anthroposophy—what was taught would only be accepted if it was also experienced as a living reality. In Emerson College itself, in the form and structure of the community and in the people they met there who carried the work, they must find a living expression of what they learned in the classroom. Students sometimes said that if they wanted just to learn about anthroposophy they could read it up for themselves in the

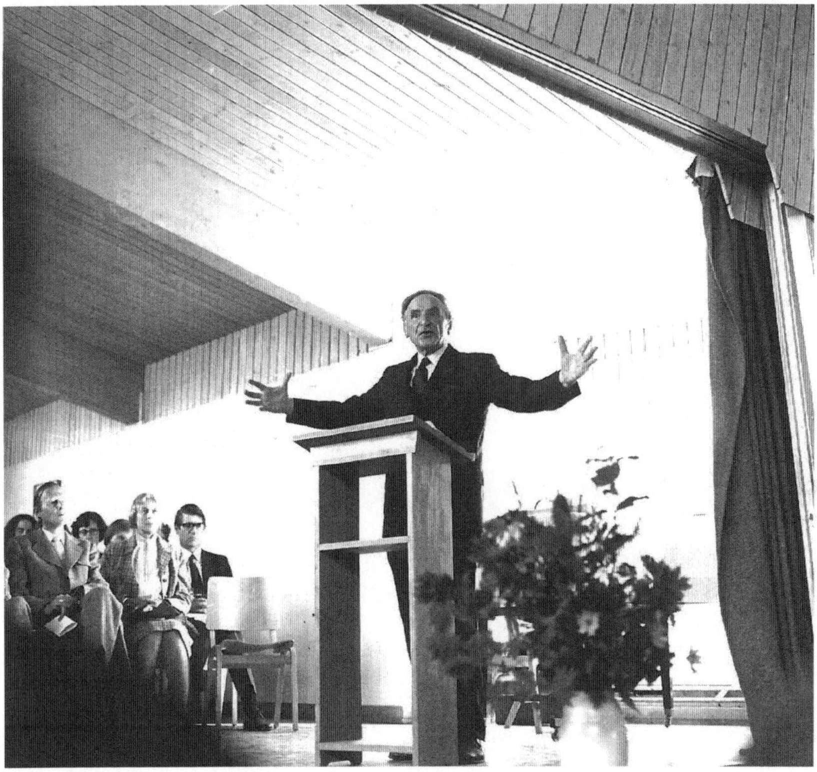

Francis Edmunds at the opening of Ruskin

library. They wanted to know what we, the staff, had made of it ourselves; how had it informed our lives and work.

Clearly, if it was to fulfil its purpose, recognition of the newly emerging individualized human being, rather than the older group soul, would have to be the basis of the community. The college would have to evolve a structure and way of working in which authority and direction came from the moral intuitions of individual people working together rather than from established forms of outer authority or conventional structures from the past. The college had to work out of what humanity was evolving towards, rather than what it should now be leaving behind in its onward development. And each student rightfully at the college should be looked upon as an individual human being in whom the future being of 'Man' willed to become manifest.

2
The Founding of Emerson College

At his funeral address published in *Circles*, the Emerson College Newsletter of Spring 1990, Georg Locher, his son-in-law, gave something of Francis Edmunds's earlier years and of his life's impulses that led to the founding of Emerson College.

> *Francis Edmunds was born on 30 March 1902 into an orthodox Jewish family in Russia. His mother died when he was only two years old, and he was brought up by his grandparents until he was about eight, when he joined his father's new family in England, where they lived first in Westcliff-on-Sea and later in London.*
>
> *Francis never spoke easily about his childhood. Already as a medical student in London he had stepped away from his family blood ties and looked to find his own independent identity and path of destiny. In his medical training he did not find the image of man he was searching for. Too young to be drafted into the First World War he nevertheless experienced suffering at the loss of young life with the deaths of young friends and acquaintances. He interrupted his studies and at the age of about 21 we see Francis in Russia as part of a Quaker relief mission, often on horseback, distributing supplies to the starving and homeless peasants. Later we see him in Beirut, among other things teaching football to Arabs, and then we see him teaching at the International School in Geneva.*
>
> *Strong inner experiences guide him to find Rudolf Steiner's Anthroposophy. He goes to Dornach, enrols in courses and meets up with the first teachers of the new Rudolf Steiner School in London (now Michael Hall). He joins the school in Streatham, arriving like a fireball with new enthusiasms and new ways. He intends to finish his medical training but the urgent need for a Class I teacher settles his destiny with Steiner's educational impulse.*
>
> *For almost 30 years before Emerson College we see him putting his immense energy and dynamism into the development of Waldorf education, as a class teacher and then concentrating on teaching adolescents in the Upper School. During the Second World War, with Michael Hall evacuated to Minehead, he writes and edits the* Michael Hall News, *founds and guides the Steiner Schools Fellowship and gives lectures to soldiers. As early as 1936 he is one of the teachers who starts the Michael Hall Teachers' Training*

Course, which started again after the Second World War and was later incorporated into Emerson College.

In the early 1950s he began his annual travels, first to America and then to the Southern Hemisphere, helping to found and develop Waldorf schools and anthroposophical groups and centres. He was a master teacher and inspirer, powerfully uniting in his work the three pillars of education: Religion, Science and Art—or as we tend to say today, the Humanities and the Sciences.

At the age of 60, after years of inner preparation, Francis was able to found Emerson College in the autumn of 1962. With his wife Elizabeth and other colleagues who joined the work he pioneered the Foundation Year, directed the Education Course and helped further courses and trainings to come into being. He wished the College with its teaching out of anthroposophy to be an adult learning community rather than an academic institution; he wished it to be strongly connected with the land, with the arts and crafts and with scientific research.

It soon became a place where the world began to meet—a world college meeting world needs, creating around the globe a human connectedness of alumni who, with what they had found at Emerson, could give new expression to their life's work on all the continents of the earth.

Francis seldom spoke of his early life. But I remember one of the few occasions that he did speak of his early years. He spoke to a small group of us of how, while he was in medical school he came to recognize that what he was being taught was not a healing of the real human being, there had to be more than just the physical body. And over against this he saw outside, soldiers marching, and it brought the picture of people at war with each other. Where could he find a true image of the complete human being, one that spoke not just of the physical body, but also of the deeper eternal soul. He went on a search for 'Man'. He felt sure that there must be somewhere a teacher, an initiate. Such a person, he felt might be found amongst the Quakers, so he worked with them. His search took him to Russia. He thought he might find what he was looking for where there was real want and suffering. Later it took him to Lebanon, and then to Geneva where he taught in a school.

On another occasion he spoke to us of how, when he was teaching in Geneva, a friend told him of regular lectures this friend was attending. Francis never joined him. Later he discovered that his friend had been going to lectures by Rudolf Steiner. He spoke of how he came to think he was not meant to meet Steiner 'in the flesh'.

★ ★ ★

In September 1961, after much deliberation and discussion with friends who recognized and understood something of the impulse that had, for many years, striven for realization within him, Francis Edmunds sent out as a preliminary announcement the plan for the founding of Emerson College. The announcement started with the following words:

A PRELIMINARY ANNOUNCEMENT

THE AIMS OF EMERSON COLLEGE

In this centenary year of celebration of Rudolf Steiner's birth, our thoughts turn also to the future, and, in particular, to the last decades of the present century. The young men and women we meet today will be the representative and responsible people then. Amongst them are many who feel an acute sense of contradiction between their intuitive regard for life and the current views, theories and events they have to meet. Their intuitions, rightly understood, may be regarded as a call for a total re-orientation of human outlook so that insights and disciplines of higher knowledge of the kind given by Rudolf Steiner in his anthroposophy may enter progressively into daily, practical life. Without this happening, the future holds promise only of growing confusion, decline and disaster, above all in human relationships which are already to be seen falling rapidly apart. Emerson College is intended, in the first place, for young men and women who have entered into their first maturity, who have completed their preliminary trainings, who may even have held office for a time, and who are alive to the need described.

Further, as the century advances, a growing onus of responsibility is seen to rest upon the Anglo-American, or, more generally, upon the whole of the English-speaking world. Communism, to which the western powers seem to be so strongly opposed, is yet no more than an aspect of western materialism raised to the status of a creed. By anomaly, it is the West, ever since the dawn of the modern age, which has nursed particularly the ideal of freedom based on the individual rights of man. In the face of this conflict, it becomes an urgent task to establish in the English-speaking West, while the times are still sufficiently favourable, whatever may give aid to those powers, designated by Rudolf Steiner, 'powers of Michael', to penetrate and to fructify western culture with new spiritual life. Emerson College will be dedicated to this task.

Finally, amongst the pernicious influences which go to shorten human vision and so to favour the spread of materialism, is the insistence in education at all levels on specialisation for limited and utilitarian ends. Emerson College will endeavour to counter this influence by engaging its students with their widely differing fields of interest in a common core of studies built on the central fact of Man, for it is in Man alone that all the diversities of human knowledge and experience find their common centre and their source. Out of a knowledge of Man renewed through modern spiritual science or anthroposophy, specialisation, too, may find its true fulfilment, namely, to lead to a higher synthesis of knowledge whereby the meaning of the world may for the first time stand revealed.

Emerson College will thus endeavour to upraise, within the hollowness of modern materialistic outlook a life-filled and life-endowing picture of Man which may truly serve as an ideal for our times, for it is ideals men need and not ideologies. It therefore takes its name from that richly significant thinker of the West, Ralph Waldo Emerson who, in his time, ever and again upheld the moral stature and the potential greatness of Man. Rudolf Steiner, out of the higher perspectives of human nature open to his spiritual-investigation, translated this ideal of manhood into practical ways of life. In striving to make this new knowledge of Man effective in thought and practice, Emerson College will, it is hoped, attain a strong and realistic place in life.

These, in brief, are the main considerations which have led to the decision to found Emerson College.

There is much in this announcement that makes it clear Emerson College would have a purpose very different from the usual sort of college of learning. In its primary task it was not intended to educate young people for any particular vocation in life. Rather it was aimed at those who had already set out in life but wished to deepen, not their ability to do a particular work, but to reach deeper into the source of their own being so as to work in the world in a way that was true to humanity as a whole and to the present time. It intended to lead young people from the very different backgrounds and specialisations in life to an experience of the all-human that is there in the depths of soul of each and every human individual. Building on the first year it was envisaged there would follow second-year courses for students intending to work in art, education, science, crafts, agriculture and nutrition.

Francis had always had a very close connection to America. He had found there people who were able to understand something of the driving force that for many years had lived within him. He had not found this recognition and support in England or Europe. While still teaching at Michael Hall he went regularly to America. Schools there turned to him for guidance and advice both in their early pioneering years of growing and in the starting of Upper Schools. In England this almost never happened.

Arising out of his connection with and support from the people of North America he thought seriously about founding the college on that continent. Many friends there encouraged him to do so and offered help. But on his return to Clent in England where his wife Elizabeth was working in the Sunfield Homes for children with special needs, he was offered by friends there space and help to found the college. For reasons given in a letter to his American friends he decided to launch the college in Clent in England. I give an extract of the letter below:

> *TO MY FRIENDS IN AMERICA*
> *At this moment of decision, my mind roams over the past nine years with its many Atlantic crossings. I think with gratitude of the many new friendships and the wonderful adventures in work which your country has given me. For me to think now of plans which might not include America seems impossible.*
>
> *The idea of one day establishing a Waldorf type of College has lived with me for a long time. I felt more confirmed in it with each passing year. The three-week student summer conferences held at the Threefold Farm were experimental feelers in that direction. It was only a question of where such a College could best be, in England or America. The very special circumstances offered by Clent, combined with the fact that I could find nothing comparable at the present time in America, finally decided me for England.*
>
> *There always were certain practical advantages to favour England. The most important are the following:*
>
> *In the first place, it is far easier to assemble the necessary teacher strength for such a College over here. Quite apart from what Clent itself has to offer, which is considerable, England being a small country and the continent being so near, additional help to make up the complement of teachers will be no great difficulty.*
>
> *Then it is far cheaper to maintain such a work in England. I estimate that, with the project for the 20 hours of practical work a week, the all-in cost for tuition, board, and European travel during vacations, comes to about $1,200.00 a year. Even allowing for the cross-Atlantic fares, this, by comparison with the cost of living in America, is very reasonable.*
>
> *Further, a College in America, on the basis of costs alone, would be confined almost exclusively to students from that continent. Here, young Americans will meet young people from many other parts, with the added*

opportunity of visiting Dornach and of gaining an impression of Europe generally.

These very real advantages will, I hope, serve to counteract the disappointment which some of you quite naturally feel that the College will not be set up in America.

On broader and more general grounds, it has seemed to me that England with its long cultural past and America with its young surging forces for the future need each other and that more could and should be done to further interchange across the Atlantic. For myself, I intend to plan the year so as to maintain connection with you all and with the work in your country—that is, if you would welcome such continued visits. Emerson College will, I am sure, thrive best if it can be considered as the child of both sides of the Atlantic. I trust that between us we can make this real.

. . . The doubt has been expressed whether American students will be ready to spend time in a College which does not grant the usual academic credits. This will certainly be a test for some, but the people I have in mind are not likely to baulk at difficulties of this kind. Credits may always be obtained elsewhere, but what Emerson College has to offer is unique. Some measure of faith there has to be that the right people will come along. I do not think it is our business to speculate too much about this. If we are convinced that such a College ought to exist, then our only course is to do all we can to bring it into being: it represents an offering-deed to our times.

This then is the burden of my present song to you. I pray it may evoke a chorus of goodwill. When I next come over, probably early in January, I will look forward to seeing many of you and we can then consider these questions further. Meantime I would like to leave you with the following thought. The Idea of the College, though I am much connected with it, should stand for itself. If it is a real idea, it will be as real for others as it is for me. It rests for each one to decide his or her relationship to the Idea and therefore how best to serve it. That way it becomes alive in many hearts. The College will be the deed of all who lend their forces to it.

I send you kindest greetings and will be happy to have your good thoughts and suggestions.

L. Francis Edmunds
1st September, 1961.

In the last two paragraphs there is an indication of certain deep truths that gave to Emerson something of its special quality and spiritual content and that made it such an important work for that time. The people for whom such a college was created would not come just because, for example, they saw an advertisement, or needed certain qualifications. A person's destiny, which carries also his pre-birth intentions, works through the will, not through thinking. As Francis often said to a student, 'It is your feet that brought you here, not your head'. Deep unconscious will forces lead us through our limbs to meet that which we need to meet. Once when we were discussing what sort of signs we should erect at the entrance to the college Francis put forward the idea, half in jest but with a serious underlying thought, that perhaps we should have an entrance that did not proclaim 'this is Emerson College', but one that was difficult to find, one to which only those students for whom the college was founded would, like Parsifal in his search for the Holy Grail, out of inner powers of intuition, find their way. Anyone who listened to the biographies of students when they related how inner questions, outer events, and circumstances led them to the college would recognize this.

In the same way on the letterhead, to give some idea of the nature or purpose of the college, under the heading of Emerson College he put the words, A College of Adult Education, based on Rudolf Steiner's Concept of Man. Nothing more. As though those who needed to find Emerson College would recognize, revealed through these words, a pointer to that which they were seeking: a place where they could find their way to a knowledge or wisdom of the human being as called for in the ancient demand of the mysteries 'Man Know Yourself'. For others the words might leave a question, or perhaps have no deeper meaning than what they appear to say.

Francis did not see Emerson as 'his' college, it was something required by the spiritual world for young men and women who, while still in the spiritual world together with higher Spirit Beings prepared for themselves a particular life's path and task. When asked the purpose of the college Francis would sometimes say that it was a place 'where young people could come to remember their task'. He sometimes also referred to himself as an instrument of the spiritual world that enabled that which was willed to come into being. I sometimes had the impression that when an aspiring student without sufficient funds applied to study at the college Francis would ask himself the question 'Is this someone for whom the college was founded?' He seemed sometimes more concerned about refusing a person who ought to be here than accepting someone who should not. Lack of funds was not sufficient grounds in itself to refuse a person, there were other considerations of a quite different nature to be taken into account.

With individual exceptions Francis would only accept students over the age of 21. He wanted those in whom the Ego was sufficiently incarnated for them to question what was presented. He thought of Emerson as a post-graduate college in that the students coming should already have been out in the world. They should have awoken to the questions presented by the world, and so to have the experience with which to find their way into what they met at the college.

The students would come along different life paths from diverse backgrounds with their individual questions and tasks ahead. They would, in their own particular ways, be people looking for a deeper reality to life than they had met in the world from which they had come. They would be looking for a place and community where they could be free to be themselves, free to decide for themselves what they would accept as true, morally good and right, and where their questioning of outer authority, including traditional and inherited beliefs, religious dogma, standards of behaviour, cultural traditions, and 'the establishment' in all its forms would be understood.

Many who came would be looking for new forms of community—for a new social order. Francis intended that students coming to Emerson would meet, in practice, in the very fabric and social structure of the college as well as in what was taught, a community of activity that was true to what humanity was evolving towards. The college must be founded on that which will be entering into humanity ever more strongly from the future, not on that which humanity had passed through and grown beyond. This meant, at the very least, that rules, regulations and an institutional structure with authority and instruction coming from above would need to be kept to a minimum. As far as possible development and guidance of the college should come from those individuals, working together, who had developed within themselves the necessary inner strengths and capacities, not from people because they had been appointed for that purpose. So too, Emerson must be a place where that which is unique and individual would be recognized alongside that which is universal and equal in all people. There must be no place for that which divides people from each other.

★ ★ ★

My impression was that Francis had an intuitive understanding of these things. His forming of the college and its social structure, human relations and administrative affairs was not something he thought through and planned in the 'loneliness of his study', but what he came to out of his years of anthroposophical study, his meditative life, and particularly to the intuitions arising out of his direct experience and observation of human affairs and, perhaps most importantly, his long experience in working with people. In the Emerson College that Francis established there was virtually no formal hierarchical structure. He himself was a modest, even a humble man. He lived modestly and drove a small car—a Mini. It was difficult to get him to talk about himself or his biography. To him that was not important. A person should be seen and valued for what he had made of himself in this life and what he had achieved, not for what he was by birth. The authority he carried was an inner authority, not one due to appointment or official position.

Fundamental to the whole life and nature of the college was the question of individual human freedom as put forward by Rudolf Steiner in his book *The Philosophy of Spiritual Activity* (now published as *Intuitive Thinking as a Spiritual Path**). It is not easy to describe what is meant by freedom in the sense meant here, but the need to leave a person free was deeply ingrained in Francis's very being. This was true in his meetings with all people, but it came to expression most strongly in his work with students. He had a real love for each one but it was not a love for what the student was as he stood there before him, but for what he saw as potential in each one, for what each could individually become. One student expressed this when she said that soon after arriving at the college she came to a sense of 'a silent expectation that each person would rise to the good that was in him or her'. She experienced this coming out of a love for each person and felt it as an enormous challenge to bring out the best. The strength of the challenge was in her being left free, experiencing no demands that she act in one way or another or believe in any given truth. Only in freedom would she come to it herself and so make it her own.

Adam Bittleston was a priest of the Christian Community based at Shalesbrooke in Forest Row where he ran the priest seminar. He also taught at Emerson College. He was a man of great experience and deep wisdom, much loved by many of the students. Many sought him out for advice and counselling. Francis valued what he could bring to the students but he insisted that when he came to the college he came as Adam Bittleston, not as a priest of the Christian Community. Adam himself understood and accepted this. For Francis it was essential that students

* Rudolf Steiner, *Intuitive Thinking as a Spiritual Path* (Rudolf Steiner Press 1995).

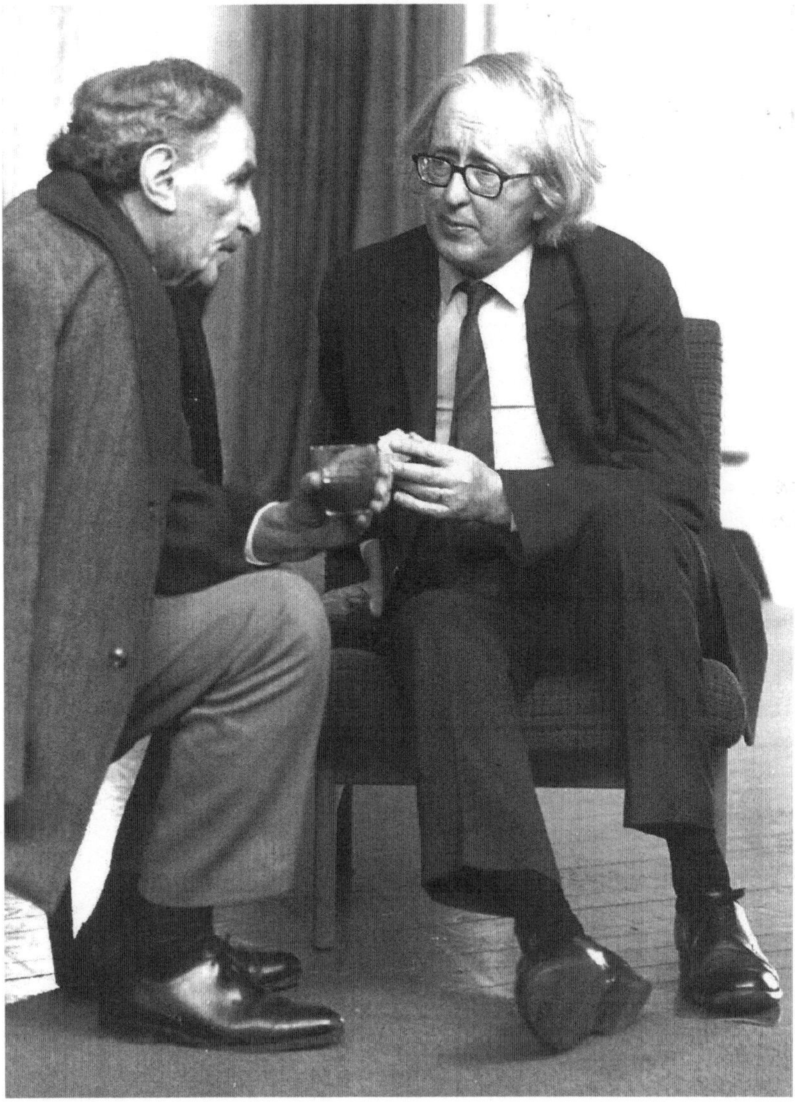

Francis Edmunds and Adam Bittleston (right)

coming to the college should not experience in any way an expectation from the college that they would or should join any particular church or religion. If they needed to find the Christian Community they would do this by meeting it through Adam as a person, not through him in an official position in the college as a priest. To Francis it was quite clear that students who had rightfully come to the college had been brought here by their karma. They had been led to Emerson in order to meet anthroposophy. An understanding of the Christ event and the Mystery of Golgotha as events that stood at the turning point of the evolution of humanity and of the Earth is at the very core of anthroposophy. This had to be presented to students quite objectively as any other spiritual fact in a way that left them free to accept it or not. This was something separate from, and not dependent on, the acceptance of Christianity as a religion.

* * *

I remember once after a particularly difficult meeting with a few of us Francis saying, jokingly but with emphasis and a serious thought behind it, that 'People are problems—if there were no people, there would be no problems!' Behind this thought was the fact that he took absolutely seriously the need to leave people free, free to unfold during their life that which they had brought with them through birth; their impulses, their destined tasks, and their particular capacities, and to come to an awakening of their own true selves. He was referring to a community of free people who, out of their own striving to awaken the good within themselves will, being human, make mistakes or take a wrong step. It is through these mistakes that a person will often come to the most important lessons in life. The teacher, the wise or experienced person, may point out a way and describe what will be found along that way, but it can only be the individual who will, facing and overcoming all obstacles, find his particular way and awaken within himself the free human spirit. He will come to this awakening only when all outer authority or direction is silenced and he finds within himself his own authority and intuitive moral guidance.

But to actually leave a person free takes courage. It requires the full acceptance of his mistakes, faults, and failings just as of his moral strength, achievements, and right actions. The world at large cannot do this. In fear of someone making a mistake or failing to do what is wanted we hedge each other round with rules, regulations, agreements, job descriptions, safeguards, and much else. We do anything but leave them free. Emerson College had to be a place where people, whether coming to study, to teach or to work in any other way, would find this freedom a reality taken right into the very social fabric of the college. Acknowledging or teaching it alone was not enough; people had to meet it in practice. Many experienced this trust in that which they bore within them as that which awoke in them a sense of responsibility.

Many of us who joined him to contribute to the work of the college came to experience, with a certain surprise, the freedom that he gave us to do the work we had taken on, whether as teachers or in the support areas of work. For myself I have been constantly surprised how he passed responsibility for much of the administrative and financial elements of the developing college to me without telling me what to do or how to do it. There was no job description. I know most of us had the same experience. Once founded, and once it became established, Francis came less and less to direct the college; he gathered people together in whom he perceived impulses and abilities and out of their united work and spiritual understanding the college developed and expanded. He continued to guide us, to ask questions, but in ways that was often a challenge to work out of the best that was in us.

However, giving freedom as he did can lead to error and create difficult problems. To allow space for something new, unplanned, and unexpected to come into being of necessity makes possible the unwanted or destructive to also come into being. People's impulses have many sources, not always directly from their karma. They often arise out of feelings and untrained emotional life. It is not always easy to distinguish between them so there has to be discrimination and courage. New creative ideas founded on one person's intuitions will not always be immediately recognized by others for what they are. Often they will be seen in a negative light. Who, for example, saw in the beginning what Francis's vision would lead to; the thousands of people's lives it would change and the good works that it would give rise to? Few of his colleagues in Michael Hall School and in the Waldorf School movement had much enthusiasm for his ideas and impulses. When he was finally ready to bring them into actual being it was mainly a few friends in America who had confidence in his vision and gave him active support. John Davy told me once that he himself had asked Francis 'Who will come to this college?' Even he could not then see that there were young people actually looking for what Francis hoped to bring into being.

* * *

On the first-floor landing of the main hall in Pixton, facing each person coming up the stairs, Francis hung a framed print of *The Polish Rider* by Rembrandt. I believe, but have not been able to confirm, that this picture also hung in the Huts.

This was an important painting for Francis; he felt that it represented something of the men and women for whom the college was founded. The picture is of a young man on horseback. The horse is moving forward to the right with his eyes clearly looking to where he is carrying the rider. The rider is looking towards the viewer but over his left shoulder into the distance. Francis often spoke of how karma and destiny work through the limbs, and in this painting he saw the horse representing the limbs—that which carries each of us through life to meet whatever lies in our destiny. The rider he saw as a consciously awakened free young human spirit, alert and interested in the world around him, and ready calmly and with courage to meet whatever tasks, events or challenges lie ahead of him in his journey through life.

3
The First Five Years

In Sunfield Homes, Clent, Stourbridge

Emerson College opened on Thursday 20 September 1962, Elizabeth Edmunds's birthday, in buildings made available to them by Sunfield Homes in Clent. Shortly after this opening of the college Francis sent out A Brief General Report on Emerson College of which the first three paragraphs may be of interest:

> *The opening of Emerson College took place on the twentieth of September, 1962. The idea of founding such a college had been long deliberated. For a time it was a question whether its home should be in America or England. Circumstances finally favoured England. Interest in its future extends to all parts of the English-speaking world and to many countries in Europe. The Founding group of students in this first year is drawn from the United States of America, New Zealand, South Africa, Norway, France and Britain. This alone shows its cosmopolitan character.*
>
> *Emerson College is intended for men and women who have already completed their normal training. The impulse behind it is not an academic one but springs from the fundamental needs related to the times. To speak of crises has become a commonplace, crises in outer events and individual lives. We face problems which no ordinary thinking can hope to solve. We propound theories which rob life of all meaning and, almost in the same breath, proclaim ideals which demand significant living. Our technical triumphs turn to moral threats. Self-determination has become a popular slogan of dictatorships. Fear is now the final argument for peace. There is a lie implicit in these things, an evasion of real issues. The moral outlook has never been more bleak. These, and many similar symptoms, provoke the feeling that something must surely end and something new begin; that there must arise a new interpretation of the world we live in, a new understanding of the nature of man. This something new can only awaken within man himself. It is in answer to this need and this situation that Emerson College has been founded.*
>
> *The college is named after Ralph Waldo Emerson, a thinker who ever upheld the ideals of the human race as evidence in man of a higher world order to which he belongs. Nor could he ever regard nature in its strength and beauty and abounding life as compounded only of the dust. Morality, not matter,*

was the basis of existence. Only he could hope to see the truth who beheld nature and human nature out of the fullness of his moral being.

The students, 11 of them, arrived the evening before the opening and entered straight into the work on the Thursday. There was no formal opening but on the Friday there was a general get-together with all immediately concerned. In January a 12th student joined from South Africa.

One of these first 11 to come to Emerson College was Graham Rickett. Everyone who came was unique and found their way along their own individual path, and what Graham says about himself gives a clear idea of the sort of paths many travelled in their search for meaning and purpose to their lives:

Starved of real substance in the various State schools I had attended, by 1960 I was hoping that, through immersing myself in the ancient language of Indian meditation (Sanskrit) at university, I might be able to combine an academic training with a meaningful path of inner development. However, the formal learning, the traditionalism and old social structures of Oxford made no sense to me, and I decided to resume my search independently on the continent.

Around that time, various books (one of them borrowed from the local public library was entitled The Philosophy of Spiritual Activity*) and magazines had come my way, which made me aware that, stemming from Rudolf Steiner's work there was an important spiritual movement centred in the German-speaking world, but active also in Britain and other countries. In 1961 I felt a strong need to establish contact with this movement, and conceived the idea of applying for a job at Rudolf Steiner House Bookshop in London.*

What I found as I browsed around in the shop was to exceed all my hopes and expectations, because there—in the year of the centenary celebrations of Rudolf Steiner's birth—I picked up a leaflet announcing the intention of Francis Edmunds to found a college named after R.W. Emerson.

The power and eloquence of the words written by L.F. Edmunds in his brochure impressed me deeply. And I was to discover later that as a lecturer he was just as much a master of the spoken word. Like Ralph Waldo Emerson the Spiritual patron of the college, Francis Edmunds placed his exceptional capacity as a speaker in the service of the impulse to overcome the materialism of the modern age and transform society through the unfolding of latent spiritual faculties. Such an inner striving was stirringly articulated in his

> *lectures, with the result that many young people, and older ones too, were inspired to dedicate their lives to the service of Anthroposophy.*
>
> *The encounter in that year with Francis Edmunds and his Anthroposophical impulse was certainly a turning point of such a kind in my own life.*

At that time the Stourbridge area, including Clent, was probably the area of greatest anthroposophical activity in the country. It included Elmfield School, Sunfield Homes, Broome Biodynamic Farm and the Goethean Science Foundation. Francis was able to call on the willing support of many of the people involved in these various activities as visiting teachers to the new college. In this way the students worked with a deeply experienced and knowledgeable group of teachers from many fields of work. For the festivals they joined in with Sunfield Homes. They also joined the staff of the Home in putting on the Shepherds' Play at Christmas. They performed extracts from A Midsummer Night's Dream, and Graham Jackson ran a choir.

Two people particularly important in the life of the college who were involved from the beginning should be mentioned here. The first was, of course, Elizabeth Edmunds, the wife of Francis Edmunds. She played an important part in the life and development of the college. By training she was a eurythmist and had a deep understanding and feeling for the reality and nature of the spiritual world as revealed through anthroposophy. It was through her that eurythmy came to play such an important part in the life and work of the college, both as an art form in the courses and as an integral part of many of the festivals. From the beginning the festivals played an essential part in the life of the community, particularly the festivals of Christmas, Easter, Whitsun, St John, and Michaelmas. Elizabeth carried the organizing of these festivals and was able to involve students in a way that was often a deep experience for them. Through her many students found their path to a professional training in eurythmy. But her artistic talents reached beyond her eurythmy as she brought art into the living and working environment of the college. While Francis enabled young people to find their path to the spirit, Elizabeth imbued the way with warmth of soul. She cared for the welfare of the students and took a deep personal interest in each one.

Lionel Elin was another very special individual. He was a deeply read and committed anthroposophist. Aged just a year younger than Francis he stepped in right at the beginning as Secretary and Treasurer. He did this out of a commitment to the idea that Francis was bringing into being. He had his own private income so wanted no salary or other support. As a young man in university Lionel had developed a severe form of arthritis due, he later told me, to travelling for some considerable distance in a train in wet clothes after playing sports. The disease effected his whole body. His spine and legs more or less completely set in a position that enabled him, with great difficulty, to hobble around, which he did with determination. When the doctors told him that he would go rigid and asked whether he preferred this to happen in a walking position or sitting, he said half-way between. That was the nature of the man. This allowed him to get around with some independence, but also to sit in a sort of leaning position. He had been like this since his early 20s. He did have rather more use of his arms and hands. In all the time I knew and worked with him I never heard him complain or dwell on his problems. He liked to be accepted as he was and treated as normal without fuss.

When the college moved to Forest Row, Lionel, and Marcia his wife, moved with it in order to continue to support the work with the young people. Marcia too was a wonderful woman. Though she herself was not particularly taken with anthroposophy she was deeply devoted to Lionel and committed her life to supporting and caring for him in every way. She was some years older than him, and told us, with a chuckle, how she fell in love with him when, not having yet met him, she first heard his deep unusual voice in the next room. This was when he was already a cripple. Her family did not approve, but she married him anyway. She started, and for many years ran, the college bookshop.

* * *

With many difficulties overcome and with others still to be resolved at the end of the first year, in his Progress Report of October 1963 Francis wrote:

> *In conclusion, when we recall the Preliminary Announcement of two years ago and the warm response it brought, and the shower of congratulatory messages at the opening of the College a year ago, and then reflect that Emerson College is no longer only at Clent, but, through its past students, is already out and active in the world, and, further, that we begin our second year with the First and Second Year Courses both in progress—when we think of all this, we must be greatly thankful. This feeling of gladness we wish to share with our many friends who, in their various ways have stood with us, and helped in thought and deed to bring all this about.*

For the second year there were 16 full-time and two part-time students. These came from eight different countries with ages ranging from the 20s to the 50s. Six of these had returned for the second-year programme.

The Move to Forest Row

During the second year it became apparent that Emerson would have to find new premises of its own. Sunfield Homes that had so generously provided space for the new college was itself expanding so, rather than being able to offer more space for the growing college, it would have less to offer. At the same time Francis was approached by the Steiner Schools Fellowship and Michael Hall School in Forest Row, Sussex with a request that he move the college to Forest Row and take the Michael Hall teacher-training course into Emerson College. They offered him buildings and land to enable him to do this. Francis had himself been active in the founding of this course in 1935 and had held major responsibility for it until 1960, so it was no foreign being that was to be absorbed into the college.

So during the summer of 1964 the college moved from Clent to its new home in St Anthony's in the Michael Hall grounds in Forest Row. This move was a major event in the development of the college. Francis describes it in his Progress Report of November 1964:

> ***A NEW CHAPTER***
>
> *Emerson College, newly installed in its second home, began its third year on the 24th September, 1964. Much preparation had gone before. A local builder and his son had been busy at work since the middle of July. The Edmunds arrived a month later. They were soon followed by a succession of students all eager to help. By the end, the place was a beehive of activity. Outside there was clipping and clearing, mowing, weeding and tidying. Inside there was painting, staining, polishing, reorganising and refurnishing of the new arrangement of rooms, and a host of other details. The result was a piece of transformation worthy of a new beginning.*
>
> *The official opening was on the evening of Friday, 25th September. Invitations had to be severely limited, yet, despite several apologies for absence over 100 people gathered in the main reception room. This fact alone suggested that the College had suddenly sprung to a new dimension. We were particularly glad to have with us Mrs. William Clark of the Steiner Educational Foundation in America; she had made the journey specially from Paris.*

There were hearty words of welcome to the students, many of whom had come long distances, and words as hearty to welcome Emerson College to Forest Row. The refreshment interval saw a great cake wheeled in with the motto: 'Welcome to Emerson College'; there followed much slicing and distributing to make sure that everyone received a share. The evening closed with a programme of chamber music. It was felt by all to have been a social festival, and much of that mood has continued ever since.

During that summer Francis also sent out a first prospectus from the college's new home. The opening statement of this prospectus pointed to a further step in the incarnation of the original 'Idea' that Francis spoke of in his letter 'To My Friends in America' given earlier in chapter 2. This opening statement was as follows:

THE IMPULSE OF EMERSON COLLEGE

Entry into the atomic age has totally altered the balance of human history. It has placed upon man responsibilities of a magnitude hitherto unknown, both with regard to himself and to his fellow-men.

The conditions which face man today are the direct consequence of his thinking of yesterday. For 400 years and more he has pursued a science based on the assumption that the world in all its aspects derives from and is subject to physical causes alone.

There are many who sense the spiritual untruth of this and the sharp contradiction it creates between the ideals they would wish to serve and the course the world is taking. Few may realize, however, that what otherwise remains in mood and feeling can, through right discipline and training, grow to knowledge and insight. Only through such knowledge, inwardly acquired, can there come the clarity and the strength to break the authoritative spell of scientific materialism. It is to young men and women who appreciate this and who seek such a training that Emerson College addresses itself in the first place.

Emerson College has thus set itself no common task. Its aim is not primarily an academic one, though learning is one of its essential goals. Rather does it wish to serve certain fundamental human needs of today. The most urgent need of all is for a concept of man, which can endow life with purpose and meaning.

The College takes its name from Ralph Waldo Emerson, a western thinker who ever upheld the spirituality at work in man and in nature. It derives its methods from Rudolf Steiner, who was able to advance the present-

day science of nature to a science of the spirit. Thereby he brought the root values of religion, art and science to a synthesis of experience within the human soul.

The result is a radical change of outlook. The key to the universe is no longer the hypothetical atom, but is man. Man is no longer a piece of highly organized matter, strangely endowed with consciousness and conscience, but a being of body, soul and spirit, significantly integrated into the world process which contains him. The separate domains of knowledge, conceived no longer peripherally but centrally through man, grow to an organic wholeness, even as the members of the body, by their very difference achieve a higher unity of being.

It is the Impulse of Emerson College to make real the thought that the ideals of truth, beauty, goodness, loyalty, love, are not subjective mental predilections, but are formative powers streaming towards man from higher sources of existence; so, too, that morality is not a code of inherited ethics, as some would have it, but is an original and ever-renewing force through which man may know himself at one with the divine. It is the purpose of the College that what is thus newly acquired in understanding shall be translated into daily action, hence the designation: 'a vocational school'.

In the two brief years of its history, 1962–64, Emerson College has drawn its students from Great Britain, the United States of America, Mexico, New Zealand, South Africa, Norway, Holland, France and Germany. The enrolment for 1964–65 adds to this quota men and women coming from Canada, Brazil, Southern Rhodesia [Zimbabwe], Denmark, Sweden, Switzerland and India. This is plain evidence that the need which Emerson College strives to meet is real and universally felt.

The buildings on four acres of land now became the new home of the college. They consisted of long wooden buildings, joined up to form a square. They had been erected before the war without planning permission by an insurance company that had then owned Kidbrooke Park. Michael Hall had used them as a hostel for their children. They were then properly known as 'St Anthony's', but under Emerson they came to be known more often as the 'Huts'. Though on Michael Hall land they were adjacent to and had their access off the Eastbourne Road so were quite separate from the school itself. The school was willing to sell the land and buildings to the college, but for the present they would be rented. When the college took them over they were old and in very poor condition. At that time the idea was to replace them with more suitable permanent buildings.

The college now consisted of a First Year General Course (later to be called the Foundation Year) a School of Education, and the beginning of a School for the Study of Biodynamic Gardening. Other schools were planned for the future. There were 26 full-time and two part-time students enrolled from 16 different countries and four different religious backgrounds. Of the 26, 16 were for the first year, nine for the second year, and one for the third year. The college was steadily growing and already becoming known worldwide. This was also demonstrated by the many visitors who attended the opening ceremony and the good wishes that were sent from far and wide.

Apart from six progress reports written by Francis I have been able to find few records for the time between the move from Clent in 1964 up to the move to Pixton in 1967. Having myself joined the college at the beginning of 1967 I experienced only the spring and summer terms in the Huts, but was at that time busy making arrangements for the move to Pixton, and so have no useful personal memory of those early years.

On moving to Forest Row a new group of supporting and visiting teachers had to be found. Michael Hall was active in encouraging their teachers to contribute to this, so Francis was able to call on many of them. Also, again thanks to Michael Hall, some of the craft courses were actually held in the school craft workshops by the Michael Hall teachers. There were also many other anthroposophists in the area who were able to bring important knowledge, skills, and experiences to the students. So the richness and spiritual nourishment for the students continued to grow.

In Forest Row Francis Edmunds himself continued to carry the bulk of the organizing and teaching work of both the Foundation and Education Courses. He dealt with all applications and correspondence with prospective students as well as the overall direction of the college. During this time he persuaded Margaret Fox to come in as his secretary (more about Margaret later).

Anthony Kaye joined the college at this time. His children had been going to Michael Hall School for some time and so he was well known to Francis and Elizabeth Edmunds. He was devoted to everything connected to biodynamic agriculture. Like many others during the summer of the move from Clent he arrived at the college offering his help. He told me later that when he had heard a tree needed to be cut down he offered to do it. But in the process he managed to nearly destroy part of a building, so Francis suggested he might help in some other way. Because of his experience in biodynamic agriculture and nutrition he then offered to take charge of the college kitchen, an offer which was gladly accepted, and so another individual came to make an important contribution to the life of the college.

John Wilkes was then a regular visiting teacher who taught sculpture. Katherine Castelliz, also a visiting teacher, lectured on biodynamic agriculture and on the Elementals. From the beginning Francis wanted all the students to make a connection with the land—to experience planting a seed in the earth, seeing it sprout and grow, harvesting it, and eating and enjoying what nature had given. Students worked their own plots, two or three to a plot. Both John Wilkes and Katherine Castelliz moved with the college to Pixton so more about them later.

Francis himself, amongst other studies, taught Parsifal, anthroposophy, botany and zoology. Other visiting teachers included: A. Heidenreich—the New Testament; Cecil Harwood—history; Olive Whicher—projective geometry; John Davy—the evolution of species; Hugh Hetherington—literature; Cecile Cope—singing; Michael Wilson—Goethean Science; Knut Ross—Bothmer gymnastics, and also Arne Klingborg from the Steinerhögskolan in Järna, Sweden, Oliver Matthews, and René Querido. William Mann taught History of Art. He was the History of Art teacher at Michael Hall and had for many years conducted trips to Italy for the Class 12 students to see great works of art. During the 1965 Easter holidays, following a request by the students, he took a party from Emerson to Italy to actually see and experience some of the works of art he had been talking about. So started the 'Italy Art Tours' for adults at Emerson. He helped arrange and gave advice for these many times during the coming years.

The second year in the Huts, 1965–66, started well with an increase in student numbers to 40. Plans moved ahead for the college to build on the site. Michael Hall offered to give the four acres. Rex Raab, an architect friend, started drawing up plans and with John Wilkes produced a model of the proposed development. Jeremy Kent also joined the college to take charge of the gardens and vegetable growing, where possible working with the students. The biodynamic course had not yet fully taken off, but some students did work with both Katherine Castelliz and Jeremy. Katherine was still involved in running the farm at Peredur, East Grinstead so continued part-time.

Though the student body had increased considerably on the previous year there was still minimal general staff to run the college. Students themselves played a major part in the organizing of some aspects of the life of the college. In autumn 1965 Francis wrote:

> *Much was accomplished in the summer months both to the buildings and in the garden to give the whole domain a new and more ordered appearance.*
>
> *Enterprise, however, went further. Some of the senior students set themselves the task of studying how the internal arrangements of the College could also be improved. It has always been understood that the day-to-day sharing of general duties, care and maintenance was an essential part of the training for future community building. The students in question took it upon themselves to take charge of all this. At the opening of the year sheets were handed out, describing the various needs and inviting students to make their choice. The Foreword read as follows:*
>
> *'The buildings which will give us shelter for the coming year need our care and attention and so does the area surrounding them. The appearance of the whole property has immensely improved since Emerson College took it over a year ago, setting its imprint on it. This good work can be continued if each one is prepared to take care of a given part of the premises. The ideal would be for each member of the College to develop a personal interest in his or her particular share of the whole, not only maintaining, but shaping and improving it, so that it becomes permeated with the workings of a human will. This way the whole College will reflect externally the life and the spirit at work within it.'*
>
> *In this way too, a load has intentionally been taken off the Principal's back, for which he is very thankful.*
>
> *In addition to these more external features, the following suggestions have also been brought forward as student contributions and are being put into effect; the planning of the Festivals, the reading of a morning verse before studies begin, grace at meals, and a regular Sunday reading of a lecture by Rudolf Steiner.*
>
> *All this is done in the spirit of service to the ideals of the College so that the character of the College may grow and develop out of the life within it, and not merely by direction from above. This way, it is hoped, each group of leaving students will have shaped something further to hand on to the new and incoming students. As an internal sign of progress, this student development is, surely, to be heartily welcomed.*

Marjorie Theyer (1965–67) wrote of this time in the Huts:

> *All the tutors were special in their own fields of endeavour. I had previously visited all the chief museums and art galleries in the western world before*

1965 but Mr Mann opened up for me what was behind all these civilisations and art works—very inspiring—also A.C. Harwood on history as a flow of consciousness. As my favourite subject at school was history and I honoured in it so all his anecdotes were wonderful. Olive Whicher blew my mind with going through infinity, Francis on Parsifal, Heidenreich on what was behind Jesus and Christ's mission, Knut was just the most beautiful human being to watch moving in Bothmer.

⋆ ⋆ ⋆

As the first new full-time teacher Mechthild Harkness joined the college in October 1966 to develop the speech and drama work.

During the three years in the Huts the college continued to grow to between 65 and 70 in the third year. The increase in student numbers had brought an easing of the financial situation, but fees still did not cover outgoings. Francis had always followed the policy not to turn away worthwhile students on grounds of finance alone. This meant that about one third of the needed fees had to be found through gifts for scholarships. Friends and supporters of the college were still meeting this need, but somehow a more assured and regular income would be needed. There was growing interest and support for the college from many parts of the world. Soon there would be a need for large donations for funding buildings that were becoming an urgent necessity. Some other solution needed to be found for running costs.

The original intention in the arrangement with Michael Hall was to build a new permanent home on that site. But towards the end of the three years it became increasingly apparent that the site offered to the college for purchase could not possibly provide adequate space for the necessary future developments. Clearly, at the rate of growth shown in the first five years, the future college, including land for biodynamic agricultural work, could not fit on to the four acres available. The resolve was then made to find another site in the Forest Row area. Much thought and activity went into this. There were a number of older mature students who became active in looking for a more suitable new home. They also made valuable contributions to the discussions helping Francis to form ideas for the future college home. These included Manning Goodwin, George and Jean Brown, and Jonathan Stedall, more of them later.

The first property seriously considered as a possible new home was Holly Hill at Coleman's Hatch. Negotiations for the purchase had progressed well until it became apparent that the assurances given by the agents that land adjoining Holly Hill would become available could not be relied upon. Francis considered it essential that the college acquired sufficient land for both a college campus and for agriculture. Agricultural land was needed for three purposes: as a base for the biodynamic agriculture course, for all students to have the important direct experience of working with nature and the growing plant, and to produce healthy food for the college. He saw that students could not develop sufficiently the necessary inner powers of imagination and discrimination on the sort of food generally available at that time. This was in the 1960s, a time of widespread materialism in the attitude to the production of food. Science had produced artificial flavourings, colourings, preservatives, fertilizers, insecticides, herbicides, and other such aids to the production, marketing, storage, and enjoyment of foods. The use of such chemicals was little questioned; they were seen as scientific advances. People who did question them were considered social oddities like the hippies. There was also little consciousness of a need to care for the environment. In his attitude to land and food production, Francis, as in other things, was well ahead of his time. He saw that the college would itself have to grow vegetables in order to provide at least some healthy nutritious food for the students if they were to work on the inner path of development which formed the foundation of the work of the college.

It was during this third year in the Huts that Roswitha and I joined the college in circumstances that themselves point to something of the particular nature of the college, so I will next give something of these.

4
Joining the College

I will explain here something of how Roswitha and I came to be involved in Emerson College, not so much because it is important in itself but because as an example it is the sort of path through which many people, both staff and students, have in their different ways been led to the College.

Towards the end of 1966, following a suggestion from my father-in-law, I had a meeting with Francis Edmunds. I was then 35 years old and was facing something of a crisis in that I had come to a kind of dead end in my life and it was imperative that I make a change, particularly in my employment. I had known Francis as a teacher at Michael Hall School where I was a pupil for two and a half years, until I was 18. I had recently come from life on a farm in Kenya. Though I enjoyed my time at the school and found it a warm human environment, I experienced the teachers mostly as a bit odd, and Francis Edmunds the oddest of all. I had no actual problems with him as a person but the feeling of a sort of barrier between us continued on the few occasions I met him after leaving school. So I was a bit hesitant to seek advice from him as to my next step. I knew I had to find a new direction in my life. I had recently come to the idea that anthroposophists would be interesting people to work with, though I was not then interested in anthroposophy itself, in fact I was probably still somewhat resistant to it. With his wide connections to anthroposophical activities my father-in-law suggested he would be a good person to talk to. So with some hesitancy I went to meet him. He had just started some new college which seemed to belong to another world.

We met in his office in the Huts. At the meeting, instead of asking me what I was looking for and how he could help, he started by telling me about the college and what he aimed to achieve. The college had now reached the point where it needed a home of its own and negotiations were well advanced to buy a property at Coleman's Hatch, the next village to Forest Row. He talked about the possibility of my coming as a student, but I pointed out the impossibility of this—I was married with two children and no money with which to pay fees etc. He then talked about my joining the staff as there was much work I could take on in connection with the estate and administration. It was an extraordinary meeting. Looking back on it from a later time I realized that within 20 minutes I knew this was my work, and this was the man I would work with and support. My life had come to the threshold of what for me was a completely new world and I stepped over it as a matter of course. I felt as though I had 'come home'. For him from the beginning it was an assumed fact that I would join Emerson College.

He then asked me what I would need by way of salary in order to take on the work. This again was a question framed in a way I had not met or thought about before. It implied a separation of salary from the work. The work was something that had meaning and value in itself, something I would do for its own sake. The salary made it possible; freed me to do the work. I experienced a reality, a truth, in this and felt completely comfortable and at home with it. He did not explain this, merely asked me what I needed and dimly I sensed what lay behind the question. At one point I even found myself suggesting I would need less than a figure he put forward, something I could not imagine myself saying in 'normal' circumstances.

The college was still in its pioneer stage of development and was limited in its financial resources. I was married with two young children. Because of the nature of the work and responsibilities I would be taking on it would be necessary for me to live on campus so the college would house me. In the employment I would be leaving I had accumulated seven years' pension rights, years that could not be replaced, and I was buying my own house in Bristol. Now I would receive less salary, own no house of my own and, for the present, no pension rights. In an extraordinary way I felt free. There would be no relationship between the work I would be doing and the salary I would be given. It was a first experience of a concept that I would build on later. He did not explain it in any way, it was simple reality to him, his way of working, and one that I came to feel as completely true to life.

When I left his office, as he accompanied me to the door I suddenly thought of something important I had omitted to tell him so I turned round and said, 'You know, I am not an anthroposophist.' 'No, no', he said, 'good, good'. He had known me at school and had met me several times since. He recognized something that I did not yet know myself; that deep down still in the unconscious depths, I was an anthroposophist.

* * *

Then I had to go back to Bristol and put it to Roswitha that we go back to Forest Row to join the pioneer staff of Emerson College. When we had married she had told me quite seriously out of deep feelings that if I ever became a teacher at a Steiner school she would divorce me. Her parents had been teachers at Michael Hall since before she was born. They were both deeply committed and long standing anthroposophists with connections to Rudolf Steiner himself. She had had anthroposophy from birth and had had enough, she wanted no more of it.

Though it was not actually taught, I had met anthroposophy in many of my teachers at school and afterwards. At that time I too, but with less reason than Roswitha, decided I wanted nothing more to do with it—I was going to lead a normal life, with normal education for my children. So, in a healthy way, we had both rebelled from what our upbringing had led us to.

So I arrived back in Bristol in a sort of state of shock mixed with excitement and trepidation. Roswitha told me afterwards that when she heard my key in the door she immediately knew a crisis moment had come. She had to make her decision; our marriage and her future depended on it. She could say 'No'. Life for her in Bristol, after five years of struggle was now going well, she had a part-time job which she enjoyed. Bristol was a beautiful and lively city to live in and we had made many friends. But she also intuitively knew at that moment that for me life would then become empty, with no fulfilment, and so something would be lost to the marriage. As she heard me walk upstairs she resolved to suppress her own true feelings and meet me with a smile, ready to agree to a move.

Looking back to that time from later years she recognized that she had made the right decision for herself as well as for me; life at Emerson brought more and far deeper fulfilment for herself as well as for me than could ever have been achieved in Bristol. But for her the first year was very difficult, particularly the first few weeks.

I then had to give notice to my employer and put the house on the market. We moved to Forest Row in early March 1967. For the first two weeks we camped in a house in Michael Hall School grounds where my parents-in-law were still active. We then moved, again temporarily, into Pixton Lodge, the mock-Tudor-style cottage at the entrance to Pixton. We were the first Emersonians to actually move onto the new campus.

5

Pixton—Finding and Preparing the New Campus

After the collapse of the plan to buy Holly Hill a group of students scoured the area for a more suitable campus. Three students in particular took on this task: Manning Goodwin, a young American entrepreneur, Jonathan Stedall, a documentary film producer for the BBC, and George Brown, an architect. Amongst other properties they were led to Pixton on the edge of Forest Row. Pixton was a large private house in its own grounds adjoining Tablehurst Farm. The owners, Jimmy and Joan Waters had previously owned Tablehurst Farm House together with Tablehurst Farm. But they had sold the house and, retaining the farm, had bought Pixton House, so joining the Pixton House property to Tablehurst Farm. Francis Edmunds had not envisaged buying such a large farm, some 230 acres, but destiny took its own course.

The Waters needed to move quickly as they wished to bid for another property nearby to be sold at auction in the near future. So a meeting was held on Friday 27 January 1967 in Pixton House in what came to be known as the breakfast room. At the meeting were Francis Edmunds with Arthur White, a solicitor, anthroposophist and friend, and his estate agent on the one side, and Mr and Mrs Waters with their lawyers and agents on the other. I understand that the meeting lasted some four hours. Jimmy Waters told me later that within 20 minutes he knew he could trust Francis absolutely, and I sensed that Francis came to the same feeling about Jimmy. I always regretted that I was not at that meeting, I was still winding down my work in Bristol.

I have always felt that it was spiritually significant that the purchase of the land and buildings that were to be the future home of Emerson College was arranged on the warm and trusting human basis that it was. Both Jimmy and Joan Waters were large and wonderful people. Physically they were both well over six feet tall and built proportionately. They also stood out in the community. He owned and ran timber businesses in East Grinstead, Forest Row, and at Sheffield Park. Farming was more of a hobby for him, not his profession, but he was at heart a country man who loved trees and the land.

The Pixton property, in addition to the main house, included a gardener's cottage, entrance lodge, coach house, and approximately 10 acres of land together with a further 40 acres of tenanted farm land. The agreed price was £35,000—fairly cheap but still quite a substantial sum of money in 1967. Tablehurst Farm consisted of some 200 acres of fairly run-down land with two sets of old farm buildings and two houses, one over 300 years old. The two properties—the farm and Pixton—ran alongside each other, though there was no easy access between them—that had to be put in later. The agreed price for the farm was £30,000, making a total with the house of £65,000.

There were two main difficulties. Francis and his supporters had not envisaged acquiring such a large farm and had neither the people nor the resources to take this on at the same time as transforming Pixton for the new college year. On the other side, the Waters needed £48,000 immediately to be in a position to purchase the farm further down the Medway Valley. So the arrangement they came to was that the college would take over Pixton immediately and pay £48,000. The college would take over the farm the following year in the spring and pay the balance of £17,000 one year later, thus solving both problems. I understand that, much to the consternation of their advisers, these two men came to this agreement within that meeting and Francis gave a cheque for the deposit. Lionel Elin told me later that after the meeting

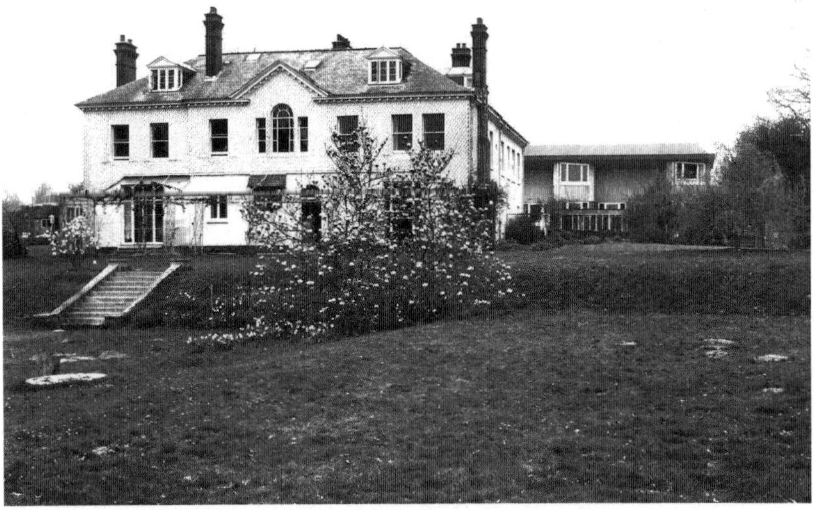

Pixton house, with Ruskin in the distance

Francis had phoned him to tell him he had just signed a cheque for the deposit and asked if there was enough money in the bank. Lionel had to do the necessary calculating and found that there was just enough.

This was a major commitment for the college. Considerably more money would now be needed to transform Pixton into a suitable campus for the college and to meet local planning requirements. A number of generous and substantial donations were received, mainly from American friends, in particular Charlotte Parker in Spring Valley, New York State, who was a long-standing friend of Francis and a supporter of his work. She contributed substantially during the early years, without her Emerson could not have developed in the way it did. There were also two other ladies in America who each gave $25,000. but I can find no record of their names.

Now began a hectic time and I had stepped right into it. An enormous amount of work had to be done if the college was to move in by the September opening of the new year. I had done nothing like this before so I had to learn as I went. It helped that I have always been of a practical nature.

The original plan was that the college would continue in the Huts for a further year and so give adequate time for the necessary alterations and improvements to Pixton. But it was soon decided to get done as much as possible in the three months available and move the college in by 25 September that year. The college would somehow cope with whatever unavoidable discomfort ensued. This, of course, put great pressure on all involved, but it was enormously exhilarating.

Pixton House, though large, could not possibly provide the spaces needed for the growing college, but there was adequate land for further building. Francis Edmunds asked an architect friend, Rex Raab, a deeply committed anthroposophist who though English practised in Germany, to draw up plans for the development of the new campus. These were to be the long-term plans, but a considerable amount of development and alterations were needed immediately. Rex found a local architect named Lambert Gibbs with whom to work. Lambert, an award-winning architect in his own right, took on the work of all the immediately necessary alterations and then later worked with Rex on the longer-term plans for the development of the campus. Pixton House itself had to be transformed from a private residence to, for the present, the main college building providing classroom space, kitchen and dining rooms, common room, offices, library, a temporary flat for the Edmunds, and later another for the Wilkes family. The coach house, in part of which was still the stabling for horses, had to be altered to provide sculpture and woodworking classrooms. The low brick-built dog kennels were transformed into a space which over the years had many uses such as maintenance, pottery, painting, smokers' common room, storage, and kitchen extension. It was a remarkably adaptable space.

For planning authority purposes and in order to give some idea as to future needs, an estimate of the number of people—students and staff—living and working on the campus had to be established. A figure of 250 was finally decided on. Based on this a new car park had to be created, a complete sewage system installed, and the road made suitable for the increase in traffic. Completion date for the purchase was not until late June 1967 so there were just three months to get all this work completed before students arrived and term started at the end of September. The builders, Durrant Brothers, were contracted to do the major work. They had to put in a complete sewage system and a car park for 65 cars. They also renewed the whole heating system in Pixton House, renovated many of the rooms and put in new flooring and widows in some attic rooms, much of which had earlier been removed. They had also to upgrade the drive and put in passing-bays. They were extremely co-operative and helpful—by the end of the summer they were pulling workmen off other building sites in order to get this work done in time. At one point they had nearly 40 workmen on the campus, in addition to our own many volunteer workers.

Also on the new Emerson campus during that summer were a large group of volunteer workers. These flocked to the college to help. They were mostly returning or new students, but there were also others who had heard help was needed and just wanted to join the work. The reputation of the college as a special place that was moving to a new permanent home was already spreading wide and many youngsters, both that summer and during many summers to follow, wanted to give their help. During that time the basis of this help was established: they came to give their work—we provided board and lodging to enable them to do so, but there was no payment, nor was board and lodging given in return for the work, but to make it possible. The two were quite separate.

We did not have proper bedrooms or dormitories for the helpers. The builders were actively going through the main house altering rooms, putting in new central heating and in some cases complete new floors, so helpers would regularly have to move their sleeping bags or mattresses, sometimes sleeping in corridors. It really was a sort of camping situation. And through it all, sometimes with builders actually working in his kitchen doing major alterations, Anthony Kaye kept the meals coming, three meals a day seven days a week, no one was allowed to go hungry. There was generally a very good mood, also between helpers and the professional workmen, with often a game of football on the lawn during breaks or, for example, a water fight between Anthony and the plumber, a large jovial man who always joined in the fun. But there were also crises and panics. Somehow we always got through those.

Roswitha and I, with our two young children, had by this time moved into what had been the gardener's cottage and the helpers often came down to us for an evening's social gathering. Roswitha regularly went to the furniture auctions in the cattle market in East Grinstead to make a beginning on acquiring some essential basic furniture for the college to supplement what would be brought over from the Huts. She also made curtains for the main windows.

At one point it was realized that there was no large room where the whole college could meet. It was decided to acquire a large wooden hut. But this, understandably, created a problem with the planning authority. They had given us permission to move to Pixton provided we demolished the huts on the Lewes Road, and now we were asking permission to erect one at Pixton. They were not enthusiastic. But as it would be put within the old walled garden—which for years had been used for chickens the housing for which was now derelict—and could not be seen from anywhere except Pixton House itself, they reluctantly agreed, but for one year only. However we did manage to get the permission renewed regularly until finally they seemed to forget about it. When Lambert Gibbs ordered the hut from the suppliers he was told 10 weeks minimum for manufacture and delivery, but he told them he wanted it in two weeks and after much persuasion they agreed. Two weeks later when it was due to arrive it was delayed and eventually arrived about midnight in pouring rain. Everyone, including Francis Edmunds himself waited up to unload it, which they did, with great good spirit in the rain and wind. Next day the builders started work to assemble it. So we got our space which for the first three years was our only large space in which the whole college could meet for festivals and the weekly house meetings. It has had many uses since then and now is an important and much enjoyed venue for the Storytellers.

* * *

About two weeks before term was due to start all the workmen were invited to join us for lunch. I remember Elizabeth Edmunds spoke the grace: 'We break this bread together, with hearts aware; not bread alone but God's life and love we share.' I remember this because one of the builders asked for the words to take home. Then Francis spoke about the college and its work. He spoke of the young people from different parts of the world, some of whom would already be starting their journey to study here. He thanked the workers for all their contributions to getting the place ready for them, but would it be ready when the students arrived?

During the last week there was an added final push to get everything finished and ready for term. All the furniture and equipment had to be moved from the old Huts to the various locations on the new campus. I remember the removal people did have a problem. They were used to moving such furniture to places which were ready to receive them, not into the chaos they found at Emerson. We were all used to it, we could see the order within the apparent chaos. But of course someone from outside would not. Even Francis, who was mostly busy in his office, still in the Huts, sometimes had a problem with it. It was unfortunate, but a humorous moment, when one of the removal men expressed himself rather forcefully while happening to look at Francis who was walking through the kitchen at the time, 'This is chaos, we don't know who is staff, who are workers who are students—talk about adult education, this is madness.' In fact it would be some weeks still before all immediately essential preparations were completed, but the college could and did start its sixth year in its new home, the new students also joining in to help to get the place finally ready.

The immediate task had been to prepare Pixton and move the college in. The existing buildings would, with goodwill, suffice for the year but were totally inadequate for the college as it was envisioned to develop. Considerable new building was required, and that would require large amounts of capital. A start with planning the necessary new building and the raising of the necessary capital were problems to which Francis Edmunds and the council of management gave considerable time and energy in the following months.

The acquisition of Tablehurst Farm would of course add to the financial pressures on the college. There was the £17,000 balance to pay in 1969. Prior to that there would be many setup and starting expenditures before it could be hoped to begin covering its own costs. Some of Francis's supporters in the USA were concerned about the purchase of the farm. They saw this as a risky undertaking that could drain money away from the college itself. At that time there was not the consciousness in the world at large of the significance of even organic agriculture, let alone biodynamic.

Francis had founded the college, not because he himself wanted it, but because out of his intuitive powers of observation he saw the urgent need for it. He was convinced such a college was spiritually required for young people of that time. It was for those who recognized this, and those who supported it, to have trust in their intuitions and go forward with conviction and courage. Courage because they could not be certain that the spiritual world would support them. Out of this trust in the future they had purchased Pixton and the farm with all that that would lead to.

6
The First Two Years in Pixton

The sixth year of the college, the first in Pixton, started on Monday 25 September 1967 in a certain amount of chaos. Space was limited, furniture still needed to be sorted out, the builders were still finishing a number of small tasks in the main house and the stairs were being carpeted. The volunteer workers, who had worked long hours in the last weeks, had either left with our grateful thanks, or transformed themselves into students. Most students and staff were finding their way around and adjusting to the new campus. This move from the rather cramped, old and deteriorating wooden huts rented from Michael Hall to the college's own widely spaced property in its own grounds was a huge change.

Some students coming from the Huts to a second year in Pixton at first missed the social quality of making do in the old Huts, finding the new home too dispersed and not yet having a centre or heart. Mary Rose Stedall was one who did. She attended the First Year General Course in the Huts and the second year Education Course in Pixton. She said the Huts had a special feel, a warm caring ambience, anti-establishment, something of King Arthur about the 'huts in the woods'. Pixton did not have that warm cosy ambience. She also spoke of Emerson being a very formative time for her, a complete transformation from her upper-class upbringing and public girl's school. Francis was of her father's generation but talked to her, and understood her at her level. He was full of vitality and his warm and caring presence was always felt.

Two other people who came over to Pixton from the Huts were John and Miriam Stevens. They both played important parts in those early days in Pixton. John was a student but also helped with the repairs and maintenance. His wife Miriam took on caring for the house. They lived in the attic where their first child was born, the first Emerson baby born in Pixton.

During the last year in the Huts there were approximately 70 students, an increase from 40 the previous year. The first year in Pixton started with around 75; 25 returning and 50 new. Of these 43 came from English-speaking countries—Great Britain 17, United States 13, Canada 4, New Zealand 4, South Africa 5, and the rest from seven European countries plus India, Costa Rica, Mexico, and Israel. There were two full-time courses: the First Year General Course; the original and much larger course later to be called the Foundation Year, and the smaller second-year Education Course.

At that time the college campus consisted of Pixton House, the stable-block, the newly erected hut in the old walled garden, and the converted dog-kennels. There was also the former gardener's house, later named Old Orchard Cottage into which, after considerable renovations, the Spence family had moved during the summer. There was a limit to the spaces available for classes and for arts and crafts. In Pixton House itself on the ground floor there were the kitchens, dining rooms, and a common room, as well as some spaces that could be used for teaching. The long dining room doubled as the main lecture room. On the first floor (American second floor) the Edmunds had moved temporarily into the west wing that had previously been the Waters's master bedroom, en-suite bathroom, and private living room. Later, when the Edmunds were able to move into their new home this became the library with the bathroom as the library office. The Wilkes family moved into temporary accommodation in the attic. The newly installed hut was the only large space where the whole college could meet for house meetings. It also housed eurythmy and drama.

Of the Emerson staff during this first year at Pixton, Francis carried the main load of the teaching as well as the main responsibility for the college as a whole, which included student enquires and correspondence. Elizabeth Edmunds taught eurythmy as well as caring for the festivals and much of the social life of the college. Mechthild Harkness taught speech and drama. John Wilkes taught sculpture but was also at that time still active in Dornach. Anthony Kaye was responsible for the catering and I for general administrative matters, finance, buildings and maintenance, etc. Jeremy Kent taught gardening and with Katherine Castelliz, still working at Peredur in East Grinstead, prepared to take over the farm in spring 1968. They were already collecting a few livestock which they kept at the back of the main house. Lionel Elin continued to do much of the accounting work; Margaret Fox was still secretary to Francis Edmunds. Roswitha Spence took responsibility for landladies and housing the students; there were then no rooms on campus. Marcia Elin ran the bookshop. Much of the responsibility for important work in maintenance, housekeeping and garden continued to be carried by individual students, often as a way of contributing to their fees.

There was virtually no accommodation for students on the Pixton campus for most of the first two years, that is, until the two student houses, with 16 single rooms, were completed in 1969. Rooms had to be found with landladies in the village. More on this later.

Perhaps here I should say something about Anthony as he played such an important part in the social life of the college in those early years. Anthony brought to the college his special qualities of warmth of soul and love of people, his commitment to anthroposophy and healthy food, and his devotion to the young people seeking anthroposophy. But his qualities of order and tidiness in his clothes and his kitchen were not such as would always delight modern health and safety inspectors. But because of who and what he was everyone ate his food and seemed the better for it. Someone recently asked me who the best cook the college had had was. I do not think one could say that Anthony was the best cook in the sense that he produced the best food. But as the one who made the kitchen into the most homely and welcoming place in the college it would be difficult to name a better one. He was always ready to help and hated anyone to go hungry. If someone was late for a meal and there was none left, instead of complaining about the lateness, he would often go back to the kitchen to find or cook something for him. This was still the case in the mid 1970s when the kitchen was cooking for up to 150 people, three meals a day seven days a week. The door to his kitchen was never locked and everyone was welcome. He also welcomed people using his kitchen in the evening. I remember often seeing Francis in there with a group of students discussing some topic of the moment over tea or coffee while someone else, for example, might be baking a birthday cake for a friend. Unfortunately early in 1978 life called Anthony back to Ireland.

At the start of that first year in Pixton most of the new students arrived on the Sunday. Roswitha had been working to find enough landladies, and now, in the college van, she met and welcomed the students at East Grinstead railway station, first bringing them back to the college to register. She then took and introduced them to their landladies. The kitchen by this time was in full operation under Anthony Kaye so meals were available for all when they arrived. It was indeed an exciting time, especially for those of us who had not previously been involved in the opening of a new year. But this time there was the added factor of it being after a hectic three months of preparation and in the college's new and own home.

At the opening meeting on the Monday morning in the Hut there was a feeling both of uncertainty and of excitement and new adventure. Francis himself seeing all the last minute chaos of the previous few days had not expected the opening meeting to actually happen, so had to improvise—which he was very good at. There were those students, friends, and staff who had been hectically working to get the campus ready and had a certain understandable tiredness about them, and there were the new students who were slightly wondering what they had arrived into, but were also happy to get stuck in to help bring final order into their home for the next year. It was actually a wonderful community-building moment. Classes started on the Monday and continued through the week, but some time was also given over to helping with a final tidying up of the college.

For many of us working at Emerson it was indeed a stimulating time. Some staff, like me, were comparatively new to anthroposophy while others had been involved for many years and had studied deeply. But Emerson was something new we all had to find our ways into. It was not an institution finished and established in its ways. We constantly had to look at the way we ordered or instituted things, into the procedures and structures. It was not enough to know how these things were usually ordered in other more established or conventional organizations. We had to understand how and why we established them here at Emerson out of anthroposophy—why we decided to do them differently, or why the same as others. The daily, weekly and termly rhythms established at Clent and through the time in the Huts continued. After breakfast when domestic duties were completed, the day would start with the reading of two verses: the weekly verse of the *Calendar of the Soul* would be followed by:

> We have the Will to Work
> Letting flow into our Work
> That which from out of the Spiritual Worlds
> Working in Life Bodily, and in Soul Spiritual,
> Wills to become Man in us.

After the first few years at Pixton, the training courses, and then later the First Year General Course itself introduced their own verses for the opening of the day within their classes. As a result fewer and fewer people attended this and it was eventually discontinued.

The college day started at 9 am to allow the domestic duties of cleaning etc., to be completed before class. This start was later changed to 8.30 am to keep in line with Michael Hall School for the convenience of students with children. With few exceptions all students and some of the staff had all meals, seven days a week, at the college. Most other staff had lunches at the college. Meals were not available with the landladies and there were no cooking facilities for students. There were mid-morning and mid-afternoon breaks for coffee or tea. In the earlier years of the college there was a long break for lunch and classes did not start again until around 3.00 or 3.30 pm. This allowed students to arrange meetings or to go shopping etc. Classes went on to around 5.30 or 6.00 pm and there were often events such as choir or extracurricular studies in the evenings. Once a week there was a House Meeting (more on these later). The cooks prepared all meals, but the preparation of the vegetables, laying of the tables, the bringing of the food to the tables, and the cleaning and washing up after the meals was all done by students. As staff numbers increased some of them joined in. These domestic arrangements, including the cleaning of floors etc., were all organized by the students themselves—at the start of the year by second-year students who handed these responsibilities over to new students sometime towards the middle of the year.

* * *

In February 1968 Margaret Shillan and Jeanne Malherbe, two first-year students, organized the first carnival. This was announced one lunch time by Hans Hager dressed in medieval costume, who rode up outside the long dining room on horseback. He dismounted and came into the room where he read from a scroll the invitation to a carnival. The carnival was to be in just about three weeks so there was not much time to get ready. I remember being amazed at the imagination and ingenuity of the students. The walls of Pixton hall were hung with paper painted to transform it into a medieval village square. The breakfast room became the Lucifer Arms and the long dining room a jousting field with the far end covered with paper painted as a reflection of the room to make it twice as long. Just off the hall was the witches cauldron. Everybody came in costume, amazingly created out of very little. The local newspaper reporter was surprised that so much enjoyment could be created without alcohol or recorded music. So was initiated the annual carnivals which through the years varied between the disastrous to the highly successful, though none have quite matched that first one.

* * *

On Monday 25 March 1968 the college acquired ownership of Tablehurst Farm as arranged under the original purchase agreement. All classes were cancelled and the whole college, together with the farm managers Katherine Castelliz and Jeremy Kent, nine calves reared on the Pixton campus in preparation, a recently purchased old second-hand tractor, and a borrowed horse and cart, went onto the new property to 'take it over'. Everyone then joined in making a start at cleaning and tidying it up. Katherine moved into the small old 16th-century farm house. The other, and newer, farm house was still occupied by a tenant and would not become available until later.

The seventh year of the college—the second in Pixton—was an important year of great change and growing up.

In addition to the First Year General Course and Education Course it had been planned to make a start with two further courses in September 1968. These would be a Biodynamic Agriculture Course and a Speech and Drama Course with Mechthild Harkness. But with the commitment of Katherine Castelliz to the initial development of Tablehurst Farm the Agriculture Course became impossible, and at Easter Mechthild had to return to Australia to take over work there.

In August 1968 Graham Rickett, who had been one of the initial 11 students in Clent, joined to take over the speech work that Mechthild had left and John Bradley, a student from the Huts, took responsibility for the repairs and maintenance of the buildings and the farm machinery. Then in September 1968 Anne Stockton joined to teach painting, Dana Prager weaving, and Peter Horsfall woodwork. Anne came from New York and brought with her many years' experience of painting and activity in anthroposophy. Her coming was also a continuation of the important connection between the college and America. Dana from Holland brought considerable expertise in all crafts connected to weaving. Peter from England came to teach woodwork in which he had developed great craftsmanship. Life later showed he had many other skills that benefited the work of the college. Later on his wife Rachel also made important contributions in a number of fields. Also joining part-time was Ann Borries who came to teach pottery and as a part-time student. She later married Roger Druitt, whom she met when he was a student, and so became Ann Druitt, by which name most people will know her, particularly for all her work later with Lifeways. More on these members of staff later.

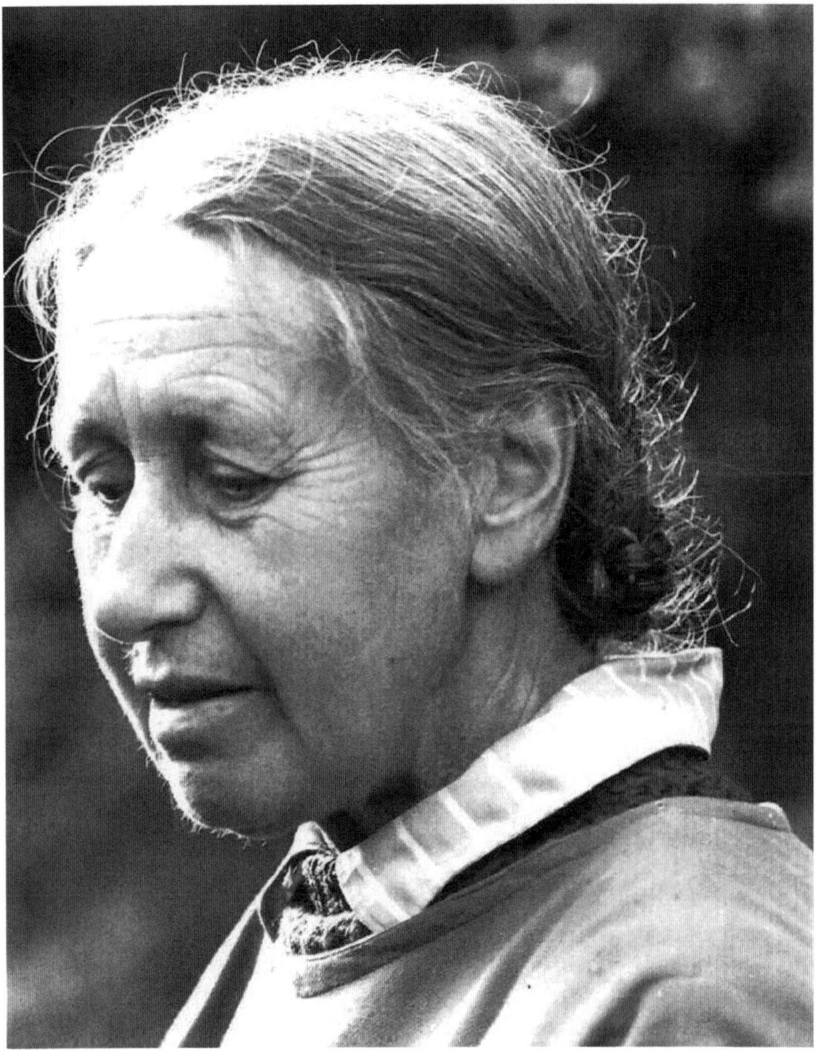

Katherine Castelliz

An important addition to the college was John Davy who joined in January 1969. Francis saw him as someone who would eventually take over from him. But John himself did not see himself in that way. He recognized that the time for leadership by a single person was past. More and more in the future we had to develop ways of working together as individuals each bringing particular insights and talents. I will be looking at this in greater depth later. In my own perception, of the two, it seemed that while each spoke powerfully to the students, Francis spoke to those questions that students brought with them through birth but which still lay in the unconscious levels of their souls, while John spoke more to those questions which had become conscious.

John Wilkes began full-time teaching in 1969 when he started the Sculpture Course. In 1970 Alfhild Wilkes began some teaching of eurythmy with Elizabeth. Walther Rudert and his wife Elli joined the farm in April 1969. He brought with him some 14 years of biodynamic farming experience and was an important addition to the leadership of the farm.

The coming of these new people to join the work had substantially increased particularly the teaching staff of the college. Up to this time Francis, with some assistance from Elizabeth, had virtually carried responsibility for, and direction of, the teaching element by himself. Apart from speech all other teaching was carried by visiting teachers. On the wider administrative side he had had much more support, including from the individual members of the Council of Management. But now with these new arrivals there could begin a sharing of responsibility for the work of the college facilitated by the beginning of meetings, particularly of the teachers' meeting. The trials of that year strengthened this carrying of the responsibility by the many.

An annual event that I believe started in the Autumn of 1968 was the International Evening. While it has always been fundamental at Emerson that individuals are primarily and uniquely themselves and cannot be defined by their nationality, they do bring with them as a sort of soul colouring something of the characteristics and qualities of the people into which they were born and lived. The idea behind the event was that early in the year, before they had lost too much of this, we would have an evening for each nationality to give something from their country, a song, story, skit or anything they liked. It could be serious, humorous or just entertaining. When this was well done the evening could give a flavour of the quality and nature of the varied cultures from which they all came.

In 1969 the first Mayfair was initiated by Ann Druitt. This came in the early summer, just as the difficulties of that year were being transformed into strengths for the future. Like the carnival, this also initiated an event that has since been held annually right up to the present. The intention was not just to do something joyful for ourselves, but also, or more particularly, for the village community of which we were in reality a part. It was too easy for the college to become separate from the village so it

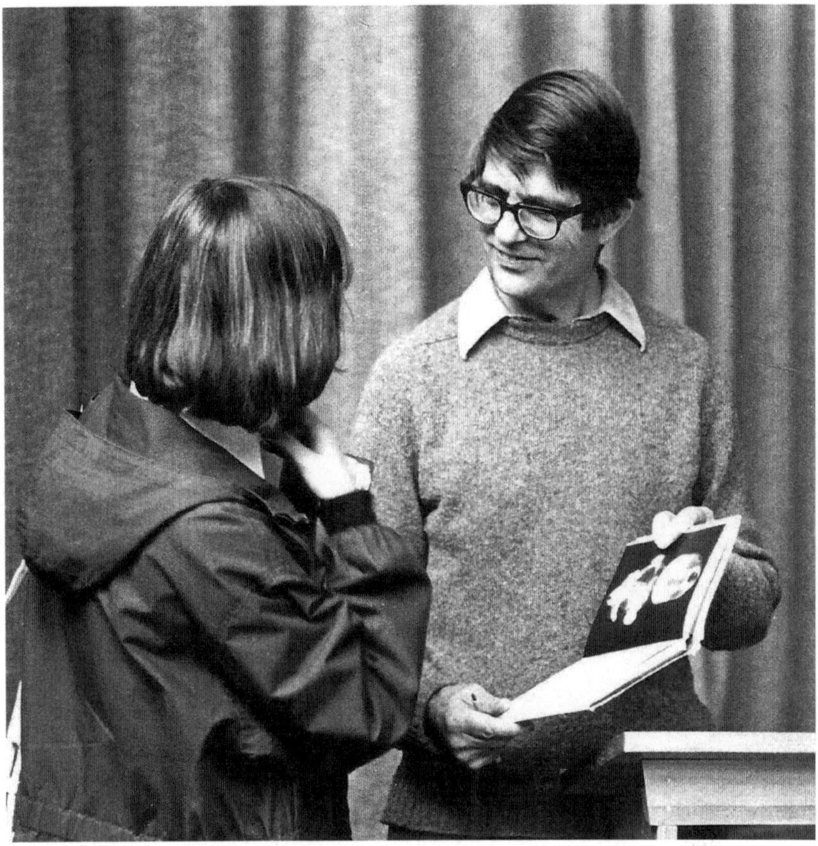

John Davy with student

was important to actually do something to reach across to the local community, to become part of it. It was also to welcome to the college the village landladies on whom at that time our very existence depended. The form of the fair evolved over the years. The focus was very much on children and nearly all children's events were free. The highlight of the event was, and still is, the Maypole dancing. Roswitha made the costumes for the dancers from sample curtain fabric books given by Rusdens of East Grinstead. The dancing was always to live music. The fact that there never was amplified music or announcements but everything was human scale gave the fair a special quality, unusual for our time. For many children this was an unusual experience obviously enjoyed. There was some money-raising for the college from the sale of tea and cakes and from stalls aimed at the parents.

The step from the sixth to the seventh year proved to be a defining one. The sixth year, the first in Pixton, seemed to bring to a certain conclusion the birth and early stage of Emerson. The seventh was often later referred to by those staff who experienced it as the difficult year, or of the year of the change of teeth. Francis Edmunds himself gave the best description of it in the Summer Progress Report of 1969. I also include the first two paragraphs as they give a good idea of the wealth of what was offered at Emerson in those earlier years. These were the visiting lecturers additional to the teachers regularly contributing to the courses.

> *This year we have further enjoyed courses by Dr. R. Koehler,. U.S.A. (philosophy), Alfred Lewers of Wynstones School (physics), Robert Kolben, Germany (music), Dr. Herbert Koepf, Germany (bio-dynamic agriculture), Arne Klingborg, Järne Seminariet, Sweden (modern art), Michael Wilson, Goethean Science Foundation (colour).*
>
> *We have also had greatly stimulating lectures by Dr. L.F.C. Mees of Holland; Dr. T. Weihs of Camphill, Scotland; Georg Unger, Dornach; Sigurd Rascher, U.S.A.; Adam Bittleston, Edinburgh; Dr. Max Stibbe, Cape Town; Mr. H.J. ten Siethoff of the N.P.I., Holland; our college architects, Rex Raab and Lambert Gibbs; and a much appreciated piano recital by Eric Harrison.*
>
> *Despite the wealth of opportunities offered, the Seventh Year proved to be a difficult one. The year began with high hopes and expectations: a notable increase in staff, a peak enrolment of 87 which later rose to 90, and, for the first time, four Schools for the Second-Year programme. By Christmas the picture was much changed. First it became apparent, mainly through the pressing demands of the work at Tablehurst Farm, that the School of Agriculture could not be maintained. Then came the announcement that Mechthild Harkness was leaving, which meant that the School of Speech and Drama must close by Easter. It further became evident that there were students who could not relate at all to the life and work and character of the College—some left soon after Christmas. and others later. Then there were students whose attitude took the opposite form—the College was not anthroposophical enough. These various elements stirred up a variety of discontents which led to much questioning as to lecturer-student relationship, the nature of the curriculum, the freedom of students to attend or not attend at will, the demand for independent group studies, the search for community—in short, questions which not without justification are being debated everywhere and which now invaded Emerson College also. The saving grace lay in the common con-*

viction that Emerson College had great potentials and in the genuine concern for these to be realized. Interpretations, however, varied greatly. Confusion seemed to increase rather than diminish. The approach to Easter was a heavy time. It was even felt and expressed that the College was going through its Easter trial, Then, from a certain point on, health and strength began to flow back again. The skies began to clear for a bright and joyous Whitsuntide. This was followed by two open days, one for the villagers, the other for teachers of Michael Hall and closer friends, both most happy occasions, with the finest display of student work since the College began. On the last Wednesday, there was an inspiring and uniting St. John's hour in the morning (we were most glad to have Dr. Rudolf Frieling with us and thank him for his contribution) and a hilarious social that same evening, full of talented surprises. The closing ceremonies on the Friday, the last day of term, recaptured all the warmth and cordiality of previous years, with the added sense that we had together suffered a chapter of trials and won through.

In retrospect much has been learned and much gained. It has indeed been a Seventh Year. Students and staff have gained a new intimacy. The life of the College has definitely reached a more conscious stage. The image of the College has taken clearer shape. Both those who stayed the year and those who left earlier may feel their contribution has in the end been positive.

7
Leadership of the College and its Meetings

Francis Edmunds tried always to work in accordance with that which was preparing in human evolution for the future, and increasingly in the future it is the individual human being that will be primary, not the group or institution. This is an essential requirement of the Time Spirit of the present—the Archangel Michael. The concept of the mission or purpose of an organization being established by the organization itself and people being employed by it to carry out that purpose may for the present have a certain justification within the economic sphere of human activity but it has no place in the cultural spiritual life of the future. It will be increasingly important that organizations such as Emerson College be formed of people who find their way to them according to their karma, or destiny. They will bring to the work those individual impulses and intentions they had prepared for the work during the time before birth. The task of the whole will unfold out of these people themselves and be formed of a working together of the individual karma, initiatives, and capacities each brings to the work.

When the college began in September 1962 it was a matter of course that Francis Edmunds who had founded it out of his intuitive perception of the needs of the time should, until there were others able to join him and share this work, guide it through the early years of its development. At that stage he was the lone pioneer and carried the full load of making all the necessary decisions with regard to the teaching, social, and administrative concerns as well as carrying much of the actual teaching. He was actively supported by a number of people, particularly Elizabeth Edmunds and Lionel Elin. But it is necessary that any such activity or organization has a legal structure. This is, in certain respects, something like the skeleton. It must be a supporting structure allowing at the same time the individual people to work and act freely out of themselves.

It was originally legally established as the Emerson College Trust, an educational Trust with Francis Edmunds, David Clement and Michael Wilson as the first Trustees. With few changes this arrangement served until towards the end of the fifth year. When later it was decided to purchase Pixton the college found itself in the position of being about to own property rather than just renting it. The Trustees were advised that it should be transformed into a limited liability charitable company.

The college was incorporated on 1 June 1967 and on Friday 14 July 1967, the first meeting of The Emerson College Trust Ltd was held, followed immediately by a first meeting of the Council of Management of the Company. The original seven subscribers to the Memorandum and Articles of Association were Francis Edmunds, Nimmo Allan, John Davy, Lionel Elin, Manning Goodwin, Ronald Jarman, and Jonathan Stedall. They formed the first members of both the Company and the Council of Management. (John Davy was unable to be at that first meeting). At the meeting the following were also elected on to the Company and to the Council: Dietrich Asten (USA), Philip Bowron, Sam Morris (USA), Michael Spence, Arthur White, and Michael Wilson. The college now had a new legal structure more suited to the tasks ahead.

Shortly before these meetings I learned from Lionel Elin that it had been decided, while I was still in Bristol, to appoint me as Company Secretary. When I asked him why I had not been consulted he was convinced that I had been. I believe he thought Francis had spoken to me while Francis thought Lionel had. This seemed to me to be another instance where one can only assume that destiny brought about a certain turn in events. If I had been asked I feel sure I would have declined. In my mind, based on my experience of the Company Secretary of my previous employment, Company Secretary was a lofty legal position where one took responsibility for the legal affairs of the company, the sort of position for someone with a degree in law. I had not even been to university and had no legal experience, though I was interested in law. So Emerson got a Company Secretary who thought and approached matters very differently than one with the necessary legal qualifications and way of thinking would have done. I do believe this made possible a certain free questioning entering into the moulding of the social structure of the college.

As I shall be using the word 'staff' very often it would be good to make clear in what sense I use it. At Emerson the word 'staff' was used for all people who carried the work irrespective of what work they did. We were all staff—teaching staff, office staff, maintenance staff, etc. Later we came to refer to each other as colleagues. This helped to overcome the division that so often occurs in many such institutions between teachers and non-teachers. I should also explain that we came to refer to ourselves as members of the Association rather than of the Company. The Memorandum and Articles of Association refers to an Association rather than a Company and, although legally we were a Company, we preferred the name Association.

The Association

Because it was a charity and would continue to be one, when the college was incorporated into a limited liability company, the authorities wished the Articles of Association to require that a majority of the members of the Council of Management (who could be thought of as Trustees) should be people not employed by, and not receiving a salary or other such benefit from, the college. But when we explained why we wanted people actually carrying the work to also carry the responsibilities they accepted this, only stipulating that no one should receive payment for the work they did as Council members, but only for the work for which they were employed. The attitude of the authorities has since changed and it is unfortunately but understandably doubtful if this would be allowed now.

This legal structure was that of an ordinary limited-liability Company with certain differences. The members of the Association were the equivalent to the shareholders of an ordinary business. Technically they owned the college, but unlike shareholders they were prohibited by law from receiving any share of the profits or in any other way benefiting from that ownership. The members of the Association elected a Council of Management, the equivalent to a Board of Directors of a business, to run the college (the business). Only members of the Association could be elected on to the Council of Management. Anyone could apply to be elected to membership of the Association but it was the Council of Management who decided whether or not to elect them. That was the legal situation.

So there were the two bodies or groups of people, one within the other: the Association and the Council of Management (the Council). The Council was formed of members of the Association elected for periods of three years. As explained above, at the beginning the members of the two were the same. The practice then was that anyone elected to the Association was automatically also elected to the Council. Another important point was that at the beginning of the new arrangement, that is, in 1967, most of the members of each were not working at or employed by the college. As originally set up, membership of the Association was for life, or until a member resigned. Members of the Association could be elected to the Council which would be for three years. The Association met every year at the legally required Annual General Meeting. This meeting would include, in addition to the formal business, a report and discussion on some issue or question affecting the work. A meeting of the members of the Association would also be called when there were important or emergency issues that needed to be discussed in a more closed group of longer serving and committed members of staff.

Later, in 1976, the responsibility and work of the Association was formulated by a committee and agreed by the Council as:

> *The Association is the ultimate guardian of the College. It is also the legal owner. It appoints a Council, to which it entrusts the formulation of general policy concerning the life and future of the College. It supports and advises the Council in this work. It also passes the accounts and fulfils such other responsibilities as may be required by the legal forms which the College adopts.*
>
> *Eligibility for Membership of the Association is open to individuals whose main work is in the College, who recognise in Anthroposophy the central source for their work, are ready to exercise discrimination and judgement on this basis, and who wish to share in the responsibilities which membership entails. Applications for Membership will usually be considered when an individual has worked for not less than two years at the College.*

Following this, in 1977 there was a major reconstruction of the Association and the Council. At that time there were some 15 members of the Association. Sixteen other members of staff were now invited to apply and were elected to membership. We then had just over 30 members on the Association—all the full-time staff who qualified, except one who did not wish to apply, and including two who were not working at the college. At the same time all members of the Council resigned and 10 members were newly elected or re-elected. From then on the number on the Council was kept to about 10, a good working number. Membership of the Association could continue to increase as the college grew.

In 1982 there was a further important development. After much discussion, it was agreed to make certain changes to the legal structure. The Articles of Association were officially changed so that members of the Association, rather than being elected for life, would in future be elected for three years only or 'so long as they worked on the premises or were employed by the college, whichever was the longer'. This meant that all those who worked at or for the college, irrespective of whether or not they were paid employees, could apply and be elected to membership of the Association. Once elected they would remain members so long as they continued to work at the college. This meant that the staff, those who actually carried the work, as members of the Association were also the owners of the college—it was their college. Those who carried the work appointed the management—the Council of Management. Others such as friends or advisers could also be elected, but then for three years, which period could be renewed. This established legally something that we had been tending towards for some time. It meant that those who worked at the college experienced themselves as also responsible for the college, they were not just employees but were also the employers. Members experienced that not only could they have a say in the selection of Members of the Council of Management, but that they might themselves at some time serve on it. The experience that we were responsible for our work, not some outside body of Trustees who employed us, was enormously enabling, freeing, and strengthening. We were the college and, more important, the work of the college was our work.

The Council of Management

This was the body legally and financially responsible for the affairs of the Association, that is, of the college. In 1967 when the new structure came into place, of the members of the Council only Francis Edmunds was fully involved as a teacher. Lionel Elin and I were both involved in finances and administration, three others were visiting teachers, and two were mature students and the rest active supporters. Over the next few years, as more teachers joined full-time, the proportion of teachers elected on to the Association and Council increased.

As the size of the Association, and therefore of the Council, grew it became increasingly difficult for it to do its business and make its decisions effectively. To alleviate this, smaller decision-making committees were periodically formed such as the Standing, Saturday morning, Executive, and Advisory Committees. Then in 1971 five members still on the Council but not actively involved in the day-to-day life expressed their feelings that they were no longer sufficiently in touch with the life of the college to be able to usefully participate in the work of the Council. They therefore resigned from the Council but remained members of the Association. So now for the first time there were members of the Association who were not also on the Council. Then, as explained above, in 1977 there was a major reconstruction of the Association when most full-time staff came on to it. At the same time within it the Council became a more distinct and smaller body with around 10 to 12 members.

It was agreed that requirements for membership of the Council should include such criteria as 'capacity to think and work out of a sense for the college as a whole', and 'has the confidence of the majority in relation to policy-making'. There was an understanding that no one represented a department but the whole had to be represented. Representing a department was not a function of membership. On one level it could be said that all important decisions that affected the running of the college as a whole were made in the Council or in one of its committees. That was particularly true with regard to the administrative and legal aspects, and it was important that this work was carried out consciously, responsibly, and competently as required by law.

Each year at the Annual General Meeting (AGM) of the Association, the law required one third of the members of the Council to resign, but they could put themselves forward for re-election. It was felt important that these should not automatically be re-elected, even if they wanted to be, but that each year there should be some change. New people should be given the opportunity to gain the experience of leadership. This would also constantly bring new life to the leadership. It was also generally agreed that there were some people who should always be on the Council: Francis Edmunds until he retired as chairman and member of the Council in 1976, John Davy because of whom and what he was, and Michael Spence as Company Secretary and Bursar. The decision to bring some regular rotation in membership of the Council meant that each year there was some actual change bringing in new members ready to take on increased responsibility. This also meant that at some time most full-time staff served on the Council. This fostered the sense that all those who worked at the college were involved in, and carried a responsibility for, not just their own particular area of work but the college as a whole.

We always tried to avoid an actual election. Over time we evolved a procedure that went some way to fulfilling the needs both of the law and of our own human social needs. Each year, well before the AGM, the work and responsibilities of the Council and the criteria for membership were discussed in a meeting of the members of the Association, or in the Staff meeting which in terms of membership, was nearly the same thing. In the early days suggestions for new members could be put to the Council by anyone. The Council would then put forward a proposal for the membership of the new Council and this would normally be agreed and voted on at the AGM. But now this was changed in that it was no longer the Council that received suggestions but a special committee newly made up each year of one member of the Council and two members of the Association who were not on the Council and who did not want to be on it for the coming year. Members of the Association could put suggestions to this committee. They would then take any suggestions from members, together with a number of other criteria, into consideration but not be ruled by them. After careful deliberation they would come to a decision who they would propose should be elected on to the Council for the coming year. This could also mean increasing or decreasing the membership of the Council. It was mutually agreed that this proposal would be accepted without further discussion. New members would then formally be elected at the AGM.

During the first years after the move to Pixton the Council met only occasionally as needed. Due to the growing amount of business over the years the frequency of meeting increased until from 1977 onwards it met weekly, usually in the evenings for about two hours. It sometimes also met on a Saturday morning to discuss matters that needed more time and to go more deeply into some issue unpressured by any ongoing business agenda. Meetings would normally start with up to 15 minutes of some form of anthroposophical study—for many years the *Anthroposophical Leading Thoughts.*[*]

The Council had increasingly become the central and final decision-making group. In its makeup it had an overall view of the whole and of the various activities within it. Most members of the Council attended the Staff and House Meetings. A majority were teachers who also attended Faculty Meetings. Although it had a core of more or less permanent members, there was regular change, so there was a feeling of the Council members as being 'us', not 'them'. In this way also the Council tended to remain 'young' and open to change and new ideas. It saw itself as carrying responsibility to both the Spiritual World and to the outer world of the State.

A Deeper Spiritual Leadership

The spiritual leadership was something acted out on a different level, not dependent on the legal or administrative structure. The Council and its committees gave a necessary structure, form, and discipline through

---

[*] Rudolf Steiner, *Anthroposophical Leading Thoughts* (Rudolf Steiner Press, 1999).

which something of a deeper spiritual nature could work but which they could not themselves provide. Spiritual leadership cannot come from a council or other elected or appointed body as such, but from individual people working together in meeting. The real leadership came from those who had made a deeper commitment to anthroposophy and who had through the necessary meditative life gone some way in developing their intuitive powers. There was at one point discussion as to whether membership of the First Class of the School of Spiritual Science should be a requirement for membership of the Council. While this was felt to be an ideal it was recognized it would also create limitations. It was important that the leadership must not become a body separate and aloof from the general life and work of the college.

There is another important aspect of leadership in our time. Occasionally in the early years, but more frequently later on, particularly when there were deep questions as to the future of the work, people would make a comment such as: 'What does the Being of Emerson want?' They had in mind, perhaps unconsciously, the picture of a Spiritual Being as the inspirer, guide or leader of the college. Such an imagination and way of thinking could have been a true one in earlier times, but now, particularly since the beginning of the Michaelic age which began towards the end of the 19th century, this thought no longer reflects the actual reality of our time. Now the responsibility to decide on a course of action, and to take the first steps on that course, has been passed from beings in the spiritual world to human beings themselves. The Spiritual World stands back and waits. Human beings can no longer wait for the Spiritual World to inspire them as to the right next action. A person must search out and decide for himself what the next right step is. This often requires confidence and courage: confidence in the way one has come to the decision as to the next step, and courage to step into the unknown; courage because one cannot be certain that this is the right next step in accordance with the will of the Spiritual World. The Spiritual World will respond, or not respond, only after a commitment has been made and the first steps taken. In such a work as Emerson College there is no guiding or inspiring Spiritual Being. Once the work has started and the people who carry the work themselves make the decisions that carries the work forward, then Spiritual Beings will join with them and support, or otherwise, their work.

* * *

The principle of not being on the Council as a representative of any particular department was an important one. A person who worked at the college was not seen through his or her particular role or function, but primarily as an individual who through his destiny brought particular impulses and capacities to the work and on that basis took on certain tasks or responsibilities. It was always important to see a person first and foremost as an individual, not as their occupation or function—we referred to people by their names, normally their first names, not their functions. They did not fulfil a job description, but, in a certain sense the description of the job and their responsibilities was built around their individual capacities and impulses, their destiny.

Many people have questioned why we did not have an outside body of Trustees as is usual with charities and now normally required by the Charity Commissioners. This requirement of the authorities is based on the assumption that people within the organization cannot always be trusted to put their own personal interests aside and make decisions solely for the benefit of the organization. From the point of view of the State this can be seen as good practice, but the spiritual world does not work through institutions of the State, but with free individuals working together in association and colleagueship. The realm of the State cannot know the power of inner self knowledge and of the moral intuitions that can be achieved by those who strive along the path of inner development in order to awaken the free human spirit within them. We are living at the time when the awakening consciousness soul is becoming active in an ever increasing number of people around the world. This means a profound change in the way human affairs must now and in the future be arranged and guided. The old forms of the spiritual world giving guidance and direction from above through a few great individuals is past. Now it must come from individual human beings working together within the community. Each brings something individual, something evolved through their incarnations as well as their resolves formed together with the hierarchies before birth. They bring these within their karma and their destiny.

The old form, that was appropriate for the group-soul consciousness, cannot now be continued by a body of expert people who, as trustees, stand outside the work, but through whom wisdom is assumed to flow and who accordingly employ, or direct, others to carry out their will. Increasingly in the future the will of the spiritual world will come to expression in those who are working together to carry out some task the purpose of which lies beyond themselves. Towards the end of chapter 10 of *The Philosophy of Freedom* Rudolf Steiner wrote:

> *For the monist, ethical commandments, which the merely inferential metaphysician must regard as expressions of a higher power, are human thoughts. For the monist, the ethical world order is the imprint neither of a purely mechanical natural order nor an extra-human world order. It is entirely the free work of human beings. Humans have to carry out their own will, not that of a being outside them in the world. They realize their own resolves and intentions, not those of some other being. Monism does not see, behind an active human being, the goals of an external world executive who determines human actions according to its will; rather, to the extent that they realize intuitive ideas, human beings pursue only their own, human goals. In fact, each individual pursues his or her special goals. For the world of ideas is expressed not in a human community, but only in human individuals. What emerges as the common goal of a human collective is only a result of separate deeds of will by its individual members, usually a few select individuals whom the others obey as authorities. Each of us is meant to be a free spirit, just as each rose seed is meant to be a rose.*

For the first seven years it was really the vision and intuitive wisdom of Francis Edmunds that brought Emerson College into being and guided it through the early years. The seventh year, as already described in chapter 6, has often been referred to by those who experienced it as 'the year of the change of teeth'. The seventh and particularly the eighth year was really the time when Francis began to pass the leadership of the college over to a wider circle of colleagues who he brought into the work: Elizabeth Edmunds, of course, and John Davy; but also people like Herbert and Ursula Koepf, John Wilkes, Anthony Kaye, Katherine Castelliz, Ann Stockton, Dana Prager, Peter and Rachel Horsfall, Michael and Roswitha Spence, and others. The future work of Emerson would emerge as the working together of the individual impulses, resolves and capacities carried in the destiny of each of these as well as others who would join this work at a later time.

Only those people actually involved with other people and able to experience, even unconsciously, what works between them out of karma and destiny will be able to come to an intuitive knowledge of how their common work should go forward, and what is needed for it. People outside can only come to theoretical ideas on the basis of a general idea of how people react to each other, not how these specific people can and do work together out of that which they each have brought through birth for this work. Rudolf Steiner points to this on different levels in several places, for example in the lecture of 9 March 1919 given in Zurich published as the fourth lecture in *The Esoteric Aspects of the Social Question.*[*]

As I pointed out earlier, Emerson College was founded just at the time when amongst many young people the consciousness soul was awakening in a powerful way. If the college was to truly fulfil its task then the students who came must find there not only the answers to their conscious questions but also, and more importantly, to meet what in a deeper sense they were looking for, a place where it was the consciousness soul itself that lived and gave form and structure to the community of people who carried the initiative. To the extent that this could be achieved the college would be quite different from any other organization or community still formed out of the old hierarchical structures appropriate to an earlier form of human consciousness.

It has also often been said that an organization such as Emerson needs people from the world at large to bring the larger picture, a business sense and practical administrative procedures to the organization. There may be some truth in this where there are no people within the institution who can translate anthroposophical knowledge and social understanding into practical organization. But it can lead to a serious and damaging division within the institution. On one side there is the good work of the teachers who base their activities on the recognition of a spiritual world and of all that arises out of that recognition, and on the other, within the same institution an administrative organization that bases its decisions and activities on widely accepted criteria of the world at large but that can actually deny the very truths on which the work is founded. In reality the structure did allow for outside advice and guidance on the Council if the need arose. There was provision for such people to be invited on to the Association. This meant that, if needed, they could also be elected on to the Council of Management. We also frequently had mature and experienced students who would ask challenging questions.

★ ★ ★

There were three other important meetings, but ones that did not have a basis in law and so were not part of the legal structure.

---

[*] Rudolf Steiner, *The Esoteric Aspect of the Social Question* (Rudolf Steiner Press, 2001).

The Staff Meeting

This was a weekly meeting for all members of staff whether full- or part-time, paid or unpaid. All were expected to attend. It was in this meeting where, more than in any other organ, something of the totality of the life and work of those carrying the college could be sensed and experienced. This was not primarily a decision-making meeting, it was too big for that. It was, in one of its functions, more of a sense organ where each of us could develop a sense or feeling of the whole. Out of this each would have a clearer idea of how any particular work was part of that whole and how to organize the work and area of responsibility so as to serve this. If a person did not attend the Staff Meeting then he or she worked in isolation from the whole.

The meeting very much evolved over time. It started as a sort of advisory group to Francis consisting of the few administrative staff before there were any regular teachers. As more full-time teachers joined the college it came to be referred to as the Faculty Meeting, although it included all staff. But as individual courses started their own faculty meetings and all staff came to the larger meeting it took on the name of Staff Meeting. Visiting lecturers and guests, particularly those from other anthroposophical institutions, would often be invited to attend. There were no clearly defined rules as to membership—these varied from time to time according to the inclinations of the current chairperson.

In one important aspect the Staff Meeting was distinct from all other meetings except the House Meeting. A member attended purely because he worked at the college. Other meetings he attended due to the nature of his work, his abilities or his particular contribution to the whole. So these other meetings tended always to divide people from each other, they separated them according to their work, their capacities or impulses, according to that which was particular in them. A person attended the Staff Meeting due to that which made him equal within the circle of colleagues, not to that which made him individual and different. An important element of this can be observed when one looks at the central task of the college. To put this simply it could be said to be the meeting of the student and the teacher. In this meeting the teacher experienced in his work the purpose and life of the college and in this his soul found inner nourishment. But where did the person in the office or doing the maintenance meet and experience this purpose for which he worked, where did he find his nourishment of soul? The final purpose of his work was indeed that the students met their teachers. But he did not experience this in his own work. Somewhere there had to be a place where that which of necessity divided people from each other was overcome, where those who made the work possible were also seen and their contribution to the whole recognized.

Only in an organization where people are able to meet each other in both these separate spheres of life, where they can meet as individuals with different capacities and different destinies but also as equal human beings carrying a common work, will there arise real community. If people come to such a meeting only for what they themselves get out of it, then something in that community of work, and in the people themselves, shrivels up and the whole work itself suffers.

The Staff Meeting was really a community, discussion, and information sharing meeting. As I pointed out earlier, most members were also members of the Emerson Association. There were occasions when what was discussed could be thought of as more properly belonging to an Association meeting. But unless there was a reason for secrecy, which there was a tendency always to avoid at Emerson, there were often advantages in involving the wider circle, rather than calling another meeting. It was a time when much information could be given: where what was happening in the courses and administrative departments, visitors expected, future events or developments, new initiatives, plans for festivals, and a review of last week's events could be shared and discussed. It was also a place where the Council could bring for a wider discussion questions or problems they were currently working on. It was important that such discussion took place before any final decision was made by the Council. In this way everyone experienced that their voice could be heard before decisions were made, that though a small group had to make the actual decisions, everyone could put in their ideas or suggestions and these would be heard.

Another aspect related to strengthening the work. We were a circle of colleagues each contributing in our own way to the college. In a certain sense we were the on-going college to which the students came. It was not chance that each one of us was in this circle; if one of us was missing there would be a gap, a break in the work. How could we really know each other, know what brought each into this circle to do the work we did if we did not meet and take an interest in each other, in who each was? Could we really do this work out of strength if we did not take a real interest in each other? What did the students gain if the staff passed each other by without interest? It was not always easy to succeed in our intentions in these areas, and there were many failings, but in many ways something was achieved. That such intentions are actively worked at is itself spiritually important.

Although, as I have said, this was not primarily a decision-making body, there were occasions when decisions had to be made, decisions such as whether we should have a Mayfair and who should organize it. The number of people in the meetings could be as many as 35, far too many to come to a decision without endless discussion. We found that the most efficient way was to have a full discussion on the question, and then ask, usually, three people who had been active in the discussion or were in some other way particularly involved, to come together, consider the question in the light of the discussion and arrive at a decision which we would accept without further discussion. The 'without further discussion' was very important, otherwise at the next meeting there would be, for example, some people who were not present at the first and had different ideas, or someone else who wanted to know why they had come to the decision. And the whole discussion would be gone through again and still no decision made.

The meeting had no permanent agreed form, but it usually started with a reading of the *Soul Calendar* verse for the week, sometimes followed by a thought or discussion. It often also included some form of study, artistic activity or singing together. There would sometimes be a review of events of the past week and of those planned for the week ahead. This could be very valuable. We would sometimes have reports from one or other colleague on aspects of their area of work. Students might also be invited in to explain and discuss proposals or areas of concern to them.

The Faculty Meeting

The General Faculty Meeting was started at the beginning of the 1983–4 academic year. The larger individual courses had had for sometime their own Faculty Meetings where they dealt with educational and administrative questions concerning their own courses. Up until then general faculty matters had been dealt with in the Staff Meeting. That had the advantage that non-teachers, who often had considerable involvement with students, could also be in the discussions. The later General Faculty Meeting met weekly and dealt with faculty matters other than those specific to the individual courses. It was also a time when teachers could share wider questions, concerns and experiences in the teaching of adults. They could work together in a common study related to their work of adult education. It was also a time to share in discussion questions as to how to help students experiencing inner soul disturbances. Practical matters such as different courses sharing the work and costs of visiting teachers could also be worked out. Students can broaden their experience of life and the world by meeting the work of other courses. Another important responsibility was preserving the anthroposophical basis of the college and maintaining this in the courses.

There were a few non-teachers who also attended this meeting. The students were adults, not children as in a school. Much of what they gained was acquired not in the classroom but in the meeting with other staff and in the general social and practical life. Some staff such as those responsible for the housing and general welfare of the students often had more insight into aspects of the soul life of students than their teachers.

Students had also to experience that both the teaching and the practical affairs of the college worked out of the same spiritual truths. The non-teaching staff needed to understand what lived in the teachers as the foundation of their teaching so as to order the practical life of the college in harmony with the educational work in the classrooms. For myself, I always felt that financial decisions and the legal arrangements should not be made in isolation from the impulses and intuitions that lived in the teachers and formed the foundations of the work. When, for example, there was a proposal for a new initiative, inevitably the question of finance, 'What it would cost and could we afford it?' would come up. If this question was asked in isolation, looking purely at the accounts, the answer might inevitably be, 'No, we could not afford it', end of discussion. Those who carry the financial responsibilities of the organization need themselves to actually experience what is working in the teachers as impulse if they are not to make their decisions purely on what is revealed in the accounts. It was always my view, and shared by others, that such decisions had to be made in meetings where those most responsible for carrying the spiritual impulse—the teachers—and those carrying legal and financial responsibility as well as being in a position to sense the movement of money within and to the college, understood and had confidence in each other. Only then could we truly work according to the spiritual conditions of our time.

It was not till late in the 1980s, after John Davy's death, that the Faculty Meeting came to be for teachers only.

The House Meeting

This was another meeting which ever since the early days in Clent played a central role in the life of the college. I look at this in more detail in chapter 13. Here I will just say that it was a meeting, somewhat like the Staff Meeting, but included all students, where the deeper impulses of both staff and students could be sensed. It was also a place where everyone could feel themselves involved in and able to contribute to the whole.

The Staff, Faculty, and House Meetings were all weekly meetings, the Staff Meeting usually around one and a half hours and the Faculty Meeting sometimes longer. They were both held in the evenings—often one before and the other after supper. It was a general policy that all such Staff Meetings, including the Council Meetings, were held outside normal class times. It often meant long working days for Emerson staff, but that was part of the commitment to the work. The House Meeting was considered part of the educational life of the college and so was usually put during the teaching day in the afternoon.

Further Thoughts

In any community there are three quite distinct spheres of activity. I would like to illustrate something of this by giving a particular example of the difference between the economic activity and the cultural life of a community or activity.

Margaret Fox was the part-time secretary to Francis Edmunds from 1966 until 1980. That was a time before computers had come into general use. It was also a time when Francis personally dealt with all enquiries and applications from potential students as well as most other correspondence. She took down all his letters in shorthand and then typed them. She also maintained the filing system. She was a wonderful woman—efficient, quick, always welcoming and friendly, and proud to be from Yorkshire. She was a long-standing anthroposophist. Her husband David was accountant at Michael Hall School, and between them they also ran a local Beginners Group—that is a group for people who wished for help in finding their way into anthroposophy. She told me once, at a time when I was myself still fairly new to anthroposophy, that from her studies of Rudolf Steiner she understood that the work she did, particularly in using the typewriter, would create hindrances to her own inner development. But she had decided to accept this as she felt that Francis's work was of immense importance to the young people of the future and this was her contribution to the needs of the time.

Margaret's work was routine and in itself uncreative. In a certain sense it was mechanical. She did what was needed of her by others, not what she needed to do out of and for herself. In this there was a separation between her inner life and her work. If she had allowed her private life, her inner soul activities, into her office work she would have found it extremely unsatisfying in that she typed letters, not out of her own creativity, but from what someone else dictated. She would not then have been able to give Francis the freedom to bring out of his own depths that which he needed to in order to fulfil his task. Rudolf Steiner has pointed out that in economic work—and her work was basically within the economic sphere of social life—a person has to let their higher abilities go to sleep. Margaret Fox understood something of this and consciously accepted it as necessary; someone had to do this work. Unfortunately this basic nature of economic work is little understood in our anthroposophical circles. Work within cultural life is quite different; in fact it has something of the opposite nature.

If a person is to join with others in the cultural work of an enterprise such as Emerson College then he cannot separate his private life from his working life. His ability to bring creativity and intuitive thinking to his work arises out of, and cannot be separated from his private life, from his own inner spiritual activity and moral behaviour. Later there were some who held that a person's private life should be no concern of the college. That may be true of those few who carried no responsibility nor wished to contribute to the spiritual life of the college, but it clearly could not be true of those who were in any way involved in the work with the students or the spiritual development of the college.

An activity or enterprise of the cultural life of human society is fundamentally different from a productive activity of the economic sphere. An electric light bulb, computer or pair of shoes is produced because other people need them, not because the people who actually make them have an inner soul-need to do so. The different and distinct natures of the three sectors of human society, that played an important part in the forming of Emerson, seem to be little understood in the wider anthroposophical community. I was deeply worried many years later when the college found itself in financial trouble due to a falling off of student numbers. Over a period a number of anthroposophical advisers were invited in to help. Much of the advice they gave would clearly have been correct and helpful to an economic productive business, but to a cultural-spiritual organization such as Emerson it could only have a deadening effect, as became apparent later on.

Though Francis continued to carry a certain vision and impulse strongly within him, he knew that all the people who came to join what he had founded, in their different ways and out of their particular lives' impulses, also brought something that would contribute to the unfolding of the work, something individual and unique that had the potential to take the impulse further into the future. John Davy too saw that leadership in the future must come from those actively involved and working together, each bringing a part of the larger idea or imagination to make the whole. Real leadership cannot come by appointment. It can only come out of the individual striving and ideas of people united in the aims of their joint work, and of their ability to recognize the contribution of each of their colleagues.

In the Progress Report of June 1970 Francis wrote:

> *Perhaps the most significant factor at the present time in the life of the College is that, whereas as little as two years ago the weight of responsibility for the work rested almost entirely on one man's shoulders, now there is a circle of men and women, united in their central impulse for the work of the College, yet greatly diversified in their gifts and abilities and carrying powers for the work as a whole.*

Francis left those whom he invited to join the staff remarkably free to do their work as they saw fit. My own experience was not unusual. As I explained earlier I came from working in a finance business. There we were told exactly what our job was and, to a large extent, how to do it. We were paid to do certain work and the employer had control over the work he paid us to do. Joining Emerson was a quite new and awakening experience, though I came to realize its full implications only later. It was like stepping into a very different world, one in which I came to sense there was a greater reality. It was my destiny path that led me to Emerson. This was my work, work I had to do out of my own life's necessity. Francis recognized this. The confidence and trust he placed in each of us itself drew that which was potential into life and being. We were not paid for the work we did, but given what we needed to meet our needs so that we would be free to do the work to which our life's path had led each of us. Most of us at that time felt something of this, each in their own way. I do not remember anyone in any of the spheres of work who came to work for the money. We could probably all have earned more elsewhere. But we all felt the urgent need and wish to contribute to this work of Emerson College.

8
The Foundation Year
(Originally called The First-Year General Course)

In the New Year Progress Report of 1984 John Davy wrote:

The Foundation Year

How do we understand this 'Foundation', now and for the future?

In the workers' school in Berlin around 1900, an apprentice asked Rudolf Steiner 'Why isn't life happier? Everyone wants so much to be happy.' 'Ah, yes,' Steiner replied, 'but perhaps our lives are not given to us for happiness.' 'Then for what?' asked the apprentice. 'Let us suppose', said Steiner 'that we have a life in order to fulfil a task.'

Thus he addressed the deep and often unconscious will with which we all come to earth. To find our individual tasks, we need to awaken to the tasks of mankind as a whole: Where have we come from? Where are we now? To what are we summoned from the future? In knowing ourselves as participants in world destiny, we begin to find the real foundations for our lives today and into the future. This, as Francis Edmunds wrote in an earlier prospectus, begins to endow life 'with grace, and purpose, and meaning'.

We know very well that anthroposophical work in the world will thrive only if it is rooted in anthroposophical life. As a preparation for serious training and commitment to one or other more specialised form of work, the importance of such a living foundation can only grow. At every turn, we see how forms of work and social organisation inherited from the past no longer hold. Inwardly, souls more easily lose their way as they meet, half consciously, the threshold trials of our times, unless they find new sources of strength and integration.

Such resources may be found in many ways. And Foundation Years of one kind or another are now springing up all over the world. What is the special character of a Foundation Year at Emerson College? And why Emerson—an American namesake for an initiative in Sussex?

While Francis Edmunds's original conception reaches back to the aftermath of the first world war, the decision to found a College matured while he was active in the United States. From the beginning, the aim was to create a centre working in the English language, which would link the old world and the new.

It is in the new world that some of the darkest shadows of our times are being met. Americans live among the rumblings of apocalypse. Yet the spiritual tasks of their world reach far into the future. The old world needs to meet and understand the drama and the real spirit of the new. By the same token, the new world needs to find roots and resources in the old.

Ralph Waldo Emerson embodies in the new world a spirit on which its true future depends. It is the same spirit which speaks through Blake, Coleridge, Wordsworth in Britain, and Goethe, Schiller and Novalis in Central Europe. They were all harbingers of a new age, prophets of anthroposophy, brought to birth by Rudolf Steiner for our times, and for all the world.

The foundation and growing up of the College in England could not have happened without the support of many Americans. American students continue to form the largest single group in the College. They join, though, a cosmopolitan community. The British Isles have given birth to the world language of today. Shakespeare, in renewing the ancient mystery dramas for the new age, forged from Celtic, Germanic and Roman sources a language for the consciousness soul which prepares for the future. This now opens doors wide to the world. There are seldom fewer than 20 nations represented in the College at any one time: most countries of Western Europe, of course; then Australia, New Zealand, Africa, Brazil, and other South American countries, Israel, India, Japan, and many more. (Will the next 21 years bring openings also to Eastern Europe, Russia, China? We can hope.)

Thus Francis Edmunds's original vision of 'a world College meeting a world need' has shown itself as prophetic. We are a meeting place for individuals from the whole world who share a search. It is a unique situation, offering access to just that sense of all-human destiny in which we can find true foundations for our lives. We are all in this together, new and old worlds alike, and need a shared foundation. In this lives the reality of anthroposophy, which Rudolf Steiner urged us to understand as 'awareness of our humanity'.

The actual forms of this Foundation Year will evolve steadily in working with those who come. We shall certainly continue to foster both Ralph Waldo Emerson and Shakespeare. But one central question unites us: How may we help the true will to awaken, so that resolves made before birth may be realised in life? In this we are all engaged in a continuing exploration and development, seeking fundamental ways for adult education which belong to the future.

The journey of the Foundation Year was a very different one from that of the second-year training courses. For those courses a student needed a more disciplined focus on the particular work he felt called to and for which he was preparing himself. His focus tended to be on a point in the future. The Foundation Year was like taking a year away from everyday life, away from the urgencies and pressures and all that constantly bombard and attack the senses, and away from looking no further than at the surface of things. It was a time to focus on the present as a starting point, and build on what the past has created to begin the journey into the future.

Francis would not normally accept students younger than 21 years of age, though he did make certain exceptions for mature younger people. In the normal development of a growing human being it is around the age of 21 that the ego enters and he felt it important that the ego was fully present when a student came to Emerson. A student had to be mature enough to question what was presented here. Francis also sometimes spoke of Emerson as a post-graduate college. By this he meant that ideally a person coming into the Foundation Year should have graduated in life. He should have been out in the world and there found the ground on which to meet and study the anthroposophy he would find at the college.

The students who joined came for many and varied individual reasons and had found their way along many different routes. Some had already met and worked with anthroposophy which had awoken in them a longing for a deeper understanding. Others had had only a brief meeting with it, but that meeting had awoken in them a deep need to know more. And there were again others who had never met it, but who carried a yearning to find answers to questions they carried deep in their souls and had been led through a friend or a 'chance' meeting to Emerson. Some knew what they were coming to, but others had almost no idea. Some could, at least to some extent, articulate their questions, in others the real questions lay still in the unconscious depths of their souls; but these would emerge often through struggle and conflict. In all who rightly came, it was possible to discern the hand of karma that at a particular time in their lives had, in diverse and individual ways, led them to a meeting, shown them a sign, or, perhaps, pointed to a book. To listen to their biographies was an extraordinary experience and a confirmation of the reality of the guiding hand of destiny and karma.

* * *

Francis Edmunds carried the Foundation Year from the beginning until 1970. He brought in many visiting teachers who made important contributions to the course, but basically he alone carried overall responsibility for the planning of the timetable and the subjects taught. He carried a consciousness of each individual student and of their soul needs as these began to unfold. He gave the main content, mainly in lecture form. Although this did begin to change as more teachers came on to the staff after the move to Pixton in 1967.

In those early years his lectures seemed to speak directly to the deeper questions of the students. Some said that they could not always remember or understand what he had actually said, but they felt they had been taken through a deep experience which lived on in them. He would speak directly to the particular students in the course. It was said that when lecturing he would know if one student was missing, even when there were 30 or 40 in the course. Francis passed over the leadership of the Foundation Year to John Davy in 1970, but he continued to carry responsibility for the teacher-training course as well as much of the guidance and correspondence of the college as a whole. He was then 68 years old. It was John who changed the name of the course from The First-Year General Course to The Foundation Year.

* * *

For the great majority of students it was a year of adventure into new territory, of questioning and initiatives, of looking into oneself as well as outwardly into the world, of challenging old customs, values and established truths, and a time to discard many of those seemingly secure guiding assumptions that inform much of social life today. It was a time to discover new foundations on which to stand, to learn what it is to be human and to know something of the long journey of evolution along which each of us has come. For many it was also the start of the journey along the path of inner development.

Over the years the Foundation Year course constantly evolved, but the greatest change came when John Davy took over the leadership. He formed a small faculty of those who carried the main ongoing teaching. He wished this faculty to carry overall responsibility for the planning, teaching, guidance, and soul care of the students; this should no longer rest with one person. Though he did not really want to be seen as the leader, due to his particular abilities he continued to be treated as such.

John was 43 when he took over. He brought to the work not only a clarity of mind and a deep wisdom founded on his scientific training, his wide interests within the sphere of spiritual science and his extensive experience of world events, but also a zest for life and a real love for young people and what he sensed lived in them as youthful intentions. Unlike Francis and many of the other teachers, John had never been a teacher nor worked in a school with children. John had been the science correspondent for *The Observer* in London for which work he had been awarded an OBE 'for services to science'. He brought with him an interest in, and an ability to connect to, interesting people and developments in the wider world. He brought his particular quality of interest in the outstanding people and events of our time not just to the Foundation Year but to the college as a whole. Although he put a considerable amount of content into his well-prepared and lucidly delivered lectures, he always encouraged students to bring their own questions as well as their own experiences and thoughts. He was a modest man who seemed always to sense that the other person also had something of value to give which he wanted to hear. He never spoke down to another person, but as one who had a real interest in the other.

Francis based much of his teaching on the story of Parsifal in order to lead students to a recognition and understanding of the moral intuitions they must come to if they were to find their way to a life based on a knowledge of the Spirit. John placed more emphasis on Steiner's *Philosophy of Freedom* and on the evolution of consciousness as a foundation for the course.

But there was always change; the students who came each year were different people with new and different questions. It was also remarkable how each year, not just the students as individuals, but the group itself expressed its own unique character, its questions and needs.

The content and timetable of the course did vary over the years, but the following is generally true, particularly during John's leadership. The first class of the day was the Morning Course. These were basically lectures, but, depending on the lecturer and the subject, could include other activities such as observation, research or discussion. The morning courses covered a wide range of subjects. Some were basic to the course and were given in some form every year. Others varied each year, depending on available visiting lecturers and also on the nature of the students of the particular year. Subjects included Parsifal with Francis Edmunds; the evolution of consciousness; man and animal; and science and technology, all with John Davy; the evolution of the earth with Herbert Koepf; plant morphology and projective geometry with Olive Whicher; karma and destiny and The Eightfold Path with Adam Bittleston; The Six Basic Exercises with Jorgen Smit; architecture with Rex Raab and others; the Word with Paul Matthews; the threefold nature of social life with Michael Spence; mathematics with Ron Jarman; darkness and light with Michael Wilson; karma and illness with Dr Mees; and many others. The students experienced that the lecturers, particularly the older visiting lecturers, brought what they did out of a love for and a wide experience in the subject. Visiting lecturers loved to work with the students, often asking for little or no payment. Morning Courses normally ran five days a week for one and a half hours up to the coffee break, and were usually in blocks of one to three weeks. They were nearly always challenging, and for students sometimes opened up quite new fields of knowledge and research.

In the Morning Course many of the lecturers were older people, often retired, who could speak out of a lifetime of experience working with anthroposophy. These lecturers were especially valued. It was intended that what was presented was done in a way that left the students free. The student could take what he had heard, relate it to his own experiences of life, and work through it in his thinking life. He would then have to decide for himself to what extent his own experiences gave it confirmation. Discussion with other students, or with other teachers, could help in this. But it could be a lonely experience. This loneliness, the experience of going into one's own thinking in order to strive towards the truth, is an important experience on the path to finding one's own true being. Ultimately a person can only know something because he himself has come to recognize its truth.

After the morning coffee break there were alternating subjects to work with in groups: Mondays and Wednesdays: study groups; Tuesdays and Thursdays: art—or the other way round. The study group is a variation on the lecture form and is generally more suitable for subjects such as *The Philosophy of Freedom* and *Knowledge of the Higher Worlds*[*] when students work directly on written content given by Steiner. It is not an alternative to the lecture, both are important and provide different approaches, neither is complete in itself. Listening to a well-prepared lecture given directly out of long life experience and then working on what has been given in the loneliness of one's study is immensely important and

[*] Rudolf Steiner, *Knowledge of the Higher Worlds* (Rudolf Steiner Press, 1969).

rewarding when working deeply into a subject. Working over a given content with others in the study group cannot replace this; it lacks the direct life experience of the individual teacher. But it is a valid and different way of working, particularly with difficult subjects. What is then worked with still needs to be taken in and meditated on in the loneliness of one's study to make it one's own. Some people find the lecture more fruitful, others the study group. The study group also fulfilled an important role as a social gathering where the students could meet, discuss and help each other on a quite different level than in the normal day-to-day meetings, not least in meeting each other's culture and language.

The study groups ran for the two hours to lunch. During the first term all students worked in small groups with different teachers on *The Philosophy of Freedom* (now published as *Intuitive Thinking as a Spiritual Path*). For most this was a difficult but immensely important study. Questions raised often continued to be discussed beyond the classroom and so set a certain tone to the college as a whole. One always knew which chapter was being studied. *The Philosophy of Freedom* was a challenge to their thinking abilities and in it they found a path along which they could strive to the awakening of intuitive and moral powers of thinking and the possibility of the birth of the higher self within them. Through moral intuitions the human being can find within himself that same source of wisdom and moral certainty that in former times was given to him from without, from what was generally referred to as God, who spoke through the prophets and the mystery centres. These study groups, out of their own choosing, sometimes ran into the second term.

In the second term, and sometimes into the third term, there was a choice of study groups offered. Subjects included *Knowledge of the Higher Worlds*, *Manifestations of Karma*,[*] *Theosophy*,[†] and *Towards Social Renewal*.[‡]

For the morning art classes the course was divided into four groups: each would do two artistic activities in two one-hour blocks per week. There would be a change over at half-term. In the second term it was usually possible to choose one artistic activity in which to work more deeply. These arts included eurythmy, speech, form drawing, and singing. In the afternoons everyone was involved either in painting, sculpture,

---

[*] Rudolf Steiner, *Manifestations of Karma* (Rudolf Steiner Press, 2000).
[†] Rudolf Steiner, *Theosophy* (Rudolf Steiner Press, 2005).
[‡] Rudolf Steiner, *Towards Social Renewal* (Rudolf Steiner Press, 1999).

drama or crafts, all of which needed more than the one hour available in the morning.

Friday between coffee and lunch was usually used to review the week's work and to look forward to the coming week, as well as sorting out any other class business.

* * *

In art the student came into a quite different realm from the morning course activities. Here he worked with that which was intended to nurture in him, above all, his life of feeling, his recognition of beauty. In eurythmy, sculpture, painting, and speech he was led to a sense of the spiritual that is always there behind, and shines through, matter.

The crafts included spinning, dyeing and weaving, woodwork, bookbinding, gardening, pottery, metalwork, batik, puppetry, costume-making, and back-stage building. More details of the arts and crafts and of the teachers are given in chapter 10. While the importance of the arts is generally recognized, the value of craftwork is not always fully understood. Both Francis and John saw them as essential parts of the Foundation Year Course for several reasons. Increasingly in our time many people reach adulthood without ever having had the joy and confidence-building experience of using their hands to create something that is both beautiful and practical. Such an educational shortcoming can leave a person in a certain way handicapped for the rest of his adult life. It leads inevitably to a certain lack of self confidence. Craftwork is also an important broadening for people who otherwise would be active wholly in their head or heart forces. It brings people into creative activity in their limbs. Amongst other benefits craftwork helps to develop practical thinking in that the process of making something has to be imagined and thought through. It also develops sensitivity to materials, textures and surfaces, and to a love of beauty in the ordinary practical things of life.

But there is another important value in craftwork. Taught in the right way it can awaken in the student a true morality, a sense for truth, beauty, and goodness. Many students have commented on their awakening, in their craft classes, to this sense of what is true and right.

The arts and crafts are, of course, closely linked. In every art, craft is necessary to bring to expression what the artist intends to reveal, and in craft the craftsperson strives for a product that is both functional and beautiful. Each calls on different attributes in the human being. In the crafts the student works more in his will forces. In crafts such as woodwork, weaving, costume-making, and bookbinding he is enabled through the use of his limbs and hands to create out of the world of matter something that fulfils its function but which at the same time in the form and quality of its making reveals, the spiritual nature of its purpose.

So each week the student worked with each of his three soul forces of thinking, feeling and willing; and in these he worked towards the three aims that the human soul strives towards: truth, beauty, and goodness.

In all of this the students, in the course of each day, would bring into activity alternately their heads, hearts, and hands. But the day related to the threefold human being also in another way. In the morning, while still dimly connected to the world of Spirit from which they had come on waking, students worked primarily with what brought their Spirit Being into activity in the lecture form of the morning course. In the arts, and also to a certain extent in the group working, they brought into activity something of their soul natures, in the crafts their bodily skills. In their experience of life in the college as a whole they again experienced a threefold quality. In their course studies they endeavoured to reach up into the higher spiritual worlds; in the social life of the college, in the festivals and meetings they experienced and learned something of what it is to be human; and in the practical domestic work and caring for the environment they reached into the kingdoms of nature.

In the Foundation Year John also established, particularly through the themes of the morning lectures, a rhythm through the course of the year. The basic themes of each of the three terms followed the rhythms of the Foundation Stone Meditation: Spirit Recollection, Spirit Mindfulness, and Spirit Vision. So in the first term the Course looked, from different perspectives, at the evolution of the human being—including evolution of consciousness, man and animal, and of the Earth. In the second term it looked more out into the world as it is today and at social questions of our time. In the third term they worked particularly with questions of inner development and preparing for future work.

⋆ ⋆ ⋆

John introduced projects into the second term. In these each student had themselves to decide on a question or theme for research, work on it during the term and present it to the class at the end of term. There was considerable freedom as to what they chose, but it was suggested that it involve research achievable within the time and practical limitations of the college and local resources (there was no internet then). They could approach any member of staff for help or guidance and they had the use of the fairly extensive college library. The choosing of a question or theme, then working out how to research it, was often the difficult part of the project. Most students, but not all, chose themes arising out of the course work, or questions they had brought with them but which had not yet found answers. Questions or subjects worked with ranged from 'Who is God?'; 'Crafting a Lyre'; to 'The Course of the River Medway'. Projects were normally individual but sometimes two or three students combined to research something together, as when three students each researched one of the three sectors of the three spheres of society. The presentations were usually made into a social event. The third term usually included studies on the architecture of the Goetheanum, the Foundation Stone Meditation, the Eightfold Path and, of course, Shakespeare.

What I have described here as the outline of the timetable was, of course, only the basic structure of the Course which varied from time to time and into which also many other events and activities were periodically added. These brought variation and new dimensions to the experience of the Course and so imbued it with life and activity. No two years were the same, just as no two groups of students were the same. Students often commented to the effect that in all these widely varied subjects and activities and in what the many different teachers brought, they constantly experienced common deeper truths that connected the different subjects into a whole.

* * *

There was no clear dividing line between the Course itself and the life of the college as a whole. In the domestic work, the washing up after meals and the cleaning of the floors and toilets, the students experienced doing something, because it needed to be done, rather than because they wanted to do it or because they personally benefited from the doing of it. To balance the Course work, which a student did because he himself out of his own inner necessity chose to do it, with work for the community that was done 'because it needed doing', is a balancing rhythm between two polarities just as necessary to a healthy inner life as is breathing in and breathing out for the health of the body. The students lived and studied in a community where what was taught in the classroom was, as far as possible, consciously or unconsciously experienced as reality in the practical arrangements of the college. Basic to the administrative agreements behind, for example, the employment of staff, the payment of salaries, and the charging of tuition fees was the recognition of what they learned in the classroom as the working of destiny and karma. This was in strong contrast to the way such matters were dealt with in the world at large from which they had come, and to which they would eventually return.

In the celebrations of the cycle of the Christian festivals of Michaelmas, Christmas, Easter, Whitsun, and St John was the possibility of experiencing a further aspect of the working of the spiritual world into the earthly life of humanity. Consciously or unconsciously, the students who came in their search for an understanding of the spiritual at work in the world, or for a path to the spirit, had been led by their karma to the Foundation Year Course at Emerson College in order to meet, or to deepen their work with, anthroposophy. At the core of anthroposophy is the change that was brought about in human evolution by the Christ event, particularly of the crucifixion and resurrection of Christ and the sending of the Holy Spirit at Pentecost. Francis always felt it right that at Emerson these events be treated as spiritual deeds that were enacted by beings of the spiritual world at a particular point in human evolution, rather than as religious beliefs. Students coming to Emerson had to be free from any pressure to involve themselves in any particular religious persuasion. These events had to be studied, in the first place, as objective spiritual facts, not as a matter of faith or religious belief.

But as objective spiritual events, the festivals could be, and indeed needed to be, approached with great reverence. They were particular times in the course of the year when we can again and again turn our thoughts and re-connect ourselves to these events which speak to us of what has been given in order that we can be free and individual human beings. These festivals raised many questions the answers to which were not always easy for students, as for many of us, to grasp, but something they could take away and live with beyond their time at Emerson.

* * *

The Christmas and Shakespeare plays were also important events though these were not originally part of the Foundation Year Course itself but were college events. The first full Shakespeare play, *The Tempest,* was put on during the summer term in 1970. From that time, until the end of the 1980s, every year in the summer term a Shakespeare play was produced with two or three performances, at least one of which was a public performance. At the beginning they were extracurricular for the college as a whole and were directed by Francis Edmunds. Though mainly from the Foundation Year, students from other courses participated. It was not until the late 1970s, after Francis withdrew from directing them, that they were taken into and became part of the Foundation Year timetable. But they had always, nevertheless, played a large part in the Foundation Year experience. Most students were involved in them in one way or other, either on stage or behind the scenes. Through Francis's directing and Roswitha's work with colour and texture in the costume-making and stage-building they met and experienced a great deal of the wisdom of Shakespeare.

As both the Shakespeare and Christmas plays played a large part in the life of the college as a whole I shall describe these in more detail in chapter 12.

* * *

Teachers on the Foundation Year Faculty, other than those already mentioned above or who taught arts or crafts described in chapter 10, who at different times made important contributions to the Course, were John Meeks who lectured on astronomy and also taught in study groups; Alistair Macdonald who ran study groups on *The Philosophy of Freedom*; Margli Matthews who covered many areas of study and lecturing and was for a period one of the main carriers of the Course; William Mann who worked with the *Manifestations of Karma*, and Carol Fraser who ran study groups mainly on meditation and related subjects. Of course after this length of time, due to failing memories and inadequate records, any listing of people cannot be exhaustive. But I think I have included all those who were with us for a reasonable length of time.

* * *

Until the end of the 1970s student numbers were never less than, but more usually well over, half the college, on some occasions up to two thirds. For the first two years in Pixton, until Ruskin was built, the course was housed in the long dining room. It then moved into the main Ruskin Hall as there was no other space big enough for it. But in reality the whole college was its space, not only because it needed so many smaller spaces for study groups and the art and craftwork, but out of the nature of the Course itself, and the students attending it, the questions being worked with tended to echo throughout the college. Ruskin was also a space used for many college functions. Even as the number of other courses increased the number and character of the students of the Foundation Year set the character of the whole. All other courses had their own rooms, but the Foundation Year called the whole college its home.

In 1967 when the college moved to Pixton there were 50 students in the Foundation Year—two thirds of the whole college. Numbers increased until in 1978–9 they reached 99. From 1980–1 Foundation Year numbers began a slow decline, while those for the college as a whole continued to rise until 1984–5. In 1979–80, for the first time, Foundation Year numbers fell below half of the whole. By 1984 they were less than one third of the whole. This change in the ratio of Foundation Year to the training courses from roughly 2:1 to 1:2 brought about considerable changes in the whole culture and community life of the college. The Foundation Year was very much a Course in which students looked inwards to come to know their own being and outwards to the world to find their way to the spirit in nature and in world humanity. They were open to new ideas and imaginations and to their own future. In varying degrees they were able to put aside the beliefs and intentions they had brought with them and were open to whatever came to them from the future. The whole community life of the college, the domestic work, the festivals, and the meeting with each other—people from so many parts of the world and with different

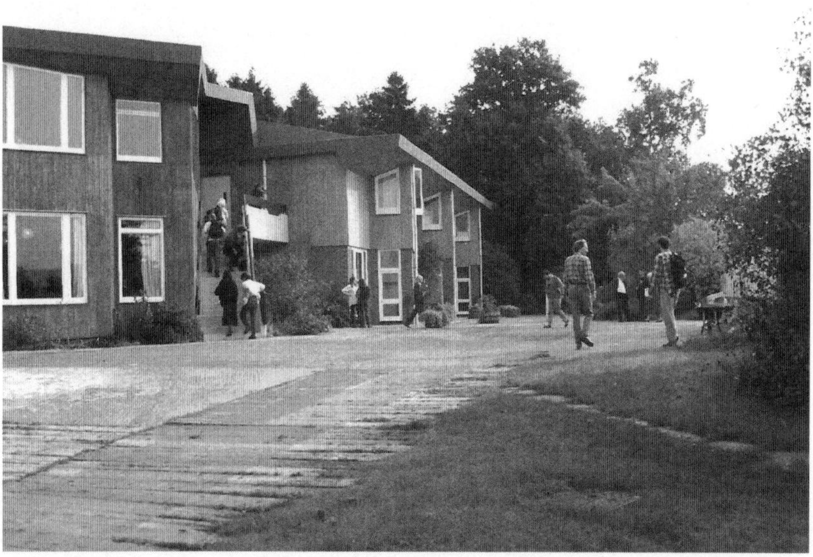

Ruskin house

destiny paths—all this enriched and enlightened their studies of anthroposophy.

But when after a year they went into a training course, the whole direction of their focus changed. Now they looked to their own particular future, to the children they would be teaching, to the land they would farm, the plant life, and the animals they would nurture, or to the artwork they would strive to create. Now they had found their future work and were preparing themselves for it. The preparation for this became urgent. They had not the same need for the community life of the whole. Domestic work often became a chore rather than something that had purpose in itself. The community life could be felt as taking time from their studies. All this was increasingly true of those who stayed on for a second and more especially a third year of training. And as the ratio of Foundation Year to the rest of the college lessened, so this different culture of the training courses began to inform the whole. I do believe that not enough attention was given to the difference in the needs and focus of a training course from that of the Foundation Year, and of the consequences for the college of this difference.

* * *

As is described more fully in chapter 20, in 1984 John developed a brain tumour, and after a short illness crossed over the threshold into the spiritual world on 28 October. But already before his illness was known he had made a start at forming a small core group of the teachers to work with him as a group in carrying responsibility for the Course. This group included Paul and Margli Matthews, John and Doris Meeks, Roswitha Spence, and Glenys Waters. When John died this group continued to carry the Course. But after a time it became fragmented. This became more intensified when, following Gideon Fontalba's visits (briefly described in chapter 21) in 1987, John and Doris Meeks and Carol Fraser left the college. Gudrun Davy then joined the group. Soon after this John Thomson was asked to join this group in order to strengthen it and, in effect, became the main Course carrier. By this time the student numbers had fallen into the 50s.

* * *

Later the Foundation Year was given its own Course room and increasingly its space and its experience withdrew from the wider college into this room. Over the years, most of the crafts slowly disappeared from the college. Looking back, I have sometimes wondered if an attempt should have been made to somehow separate the training courses more fully from the Foundation Year, giving each their own space, their own community life within a whole. That would not have been easy, perhaps impossible. It would also have created other problems. But something was lost from the impulse of the Foundation Year when the training courses grew to play an ever larger part in the life of the college—something of the experience of adventure in the Course seemed to have gone.

9
The Training Courses

In the New Year Progress Report of 1984 John Davy wrote on the training courses:

> *As the Foundation Year is concerned to awaken the will for life, so the training courses are concerned with the will for work. What is the aim of a teacher-training course? 'Not to give would-be teachers a seminar of some sort of standardised education that prescribes dogmas, but to give them the sort of thing that makes them become teachers. . . . The educator has to be born in person'. Thus Rudolf Steiner in 1920. So we are concerned with awakening the will for teaching, farming, social work, for bringing the arts into life.*
>
> *The world's needs are obvious and urgent. During the coming years, our training courses must develop in vigour and depth. It will not be enough merely to supplement orthodox trainings obtained elsewhere. While these may have various virtues—they are often replete with information and adept in various methodologies—they are seldom concerned to awaken the creative will. Indeed they often seem designed to discourage it. We must aim, in time, to develop possibilities of full trainings in all the fields where we have experience and resources.*

I will not go into the detail in describing these training courses as I did with the Foundation Year, that would take me beyond the scope and purpose of this book.

The Education Course

As described earlier, Francis had founded the Michael Hall teacher-training course in 1936 and had continued to carry it until 1960, so when it was absorbed into Emerson in 1964 he was picking up something he had long been involved with. Francis now ran this Course in addition to continuing to carry the Foundation Year, but with considerable input from Michael Hall teachers as well as others from elsewhere. Without their support the college could not have survived as there were no full-time teachers at Emerson, other than Francis, until after the move to Pixton. Even then it continued to depend on visiting teachers in both the Foundation and Education Courses.

After handing the leadership of the Foundation Year to John Davy in 1970 Francis concentrated on the Education Course, as well as overseeing much of the general affairs of the college. Numbers fluctuated, varying from 13 to a more usual number in the 30s and sometimes into the 40s.

In 1972 Ron Jarman, who was a teacher at Michael Hall and had been a frequent contributor to the Course, was invited to increase his work to half-time and to support Francis in the leadership of the Course. One factor in this was that it was now over 10 years since Francis had been engaged in working directly with children. Then in January 1975 Ron gave up his other commitments at Michael Hall and the Steiner Schools Fellowship and increased his commitment to full-time. Francis handed over main responsibility for the Education Course to him and so was finally able to withdraw from all Course carrying. Francis was then 74 years old.

Georg Locher and Margaret Shillan, both teachers at Michael Hall, had also for some years been teaching part-time on the Education Course. They now worked with Ron who continued to carry main responsibility until 1980 when he left to take on other work in the Steiner Schools Fellowship. Georg Locher had been a pupil at Michael Hall and later attended the earlier Michael Hall teacher-training course under Francis Edmunds, following which he became a class teacher at the school. He had been involved with the Education Course at Emerson for some years, but now increased his commitment.

Before attending the Foundation Year during 1967–8, Margaret Shillan had trained as a graphic artist. She completed the Education Course in 1968–9 and then, in 1969–70 worked with John Wilkes as a sort of extended Education Course before going to Michael Hall where she taught painting in the Upper School for some 15 years.

By 1977–8 student numbers in the Course had reached well into the 40s. Due particularly to the necessity for the students going for observation and practice-teaching to the various schools, both in the UK and abroad, there was a growing need for both administrative and Course work help. Lee Sturgeon, Bill Day, Elizabeth Webster, Lesley Cox, and Francesca Josephson all helped with this at different times. In 1978 the Course moved into the room that had previously housed the weaving, a space much more suitable, both artistically and socially, for their work. At that time they also began to form their own weekly Faculty Meeting. Molly von Heider and Coen van Houten, also contributors to the Course, were part of this meeting.

After Ron Jarman left in 1980 there was a year during which there was no full-time teacher carrying the Course. Georg and Margaret, together with Lesley and other assistance from the Social Development Centre, took overall responsibility for the year. Already for the year 1980–1 student numbers had fallen well below the 40 of the year before, and in 1981–2 fell to just 12. John Thomson, a class teacher at Elmfield Waldorf School in Stourbridge with many years' classroom and Waldorf school experience, was then invited to join the college. He joined at Easter 1981 and, with Margaret and Georg took over main responsibility for the Course. Both Georg and Margaret, now full-time at Emerson, were also teaching in other courses. In 1982–3 student numbers were up to 35 and by 1984–5 back into the 40s. From 1986–7 numbers again began a slow and continuing decline.

Although this was an Emerson Course it could not have run successfully without the continuing and considerable assistance given by Michael Hall School in particular, but also by the other Waldorf schools in Great Britain. During the year the students had to have regular periods in the classroom with children; generally three weeks observation in the first term and four weeks' practice-teaching in the second term. This placed an enormous burden on the schools which they continued to give despite the fact that the majority of students were from abroad and most would return to teach in schools in their own countries. The Steiner Schools Fellowship also gave important financial support.

The need to extend the Course to a three-year training was often raised. But few students could afford three, or even two, years in addition to the Foundation Year. There were attempts to bring some teacher-training modules into the Foundation Year and treat it as a first year of the education training. But there were difficulties to this and it did not really work. The Course did bring a quality of disciplined commitment to the college which was in strong contrast to the sometimes sanguine openness and excitement of what for many was the opening up of a new world in the Foundation Year. Now they quickly became more focused in preparing for their work in the future and on the children who would soon be their pupils and for whom they would carry great responsibility. They also made important contributions to the life of the college, particularly with their Advent Festivals and their contributions to the Christmas plays. More of these later.

A delightful story from Sybille Diena (Umbreit) about Francis Edmunds's lecturing:

One morning lecture, (on the role of the class teacher) Francis looked very carefully at everybody's attire and said (not in these exact words but pretty much like it):

*'As a class teacher you have ALWAYS to make sure that your appearance is as well groomed and beautiful as possible; no drooping darned stockings, no ill-fitting dress, no worn out shoes, trailing laces, loose threads, no tousled hair, unshaven stubble, missing shirt buttons, stains, patches or dirty fingernails!' And he continued with a sincere look: 'An unkempt appearance damages the ether body of your pupils! Never forget that, especially in the first years of lower school! So wear your weird stuff to church on Sunday, the Lord will not take offence—**but wear your Sunday best when you stand in front of your class!!!'***

The Biodynamic Agriculture Course

As explained earlier, Francis had intended from the beginning that there should be both an Education Course and a Biodynamic Agriculture Course. In Clent and in the Huts there had been some agricultural and horticultural studies, but the early attempts to start an actual Course had been unsuccessful. He often spoke of how he saw the farmer and the teacher as two pillars of human community in the wider sense. The third was the doctor. He had hoped to develop some sort of medical work at the college, but the right person or people to develop it never appeared.

In 1968, shortly after the move to Pixton and the acquisition of Tablehurst Farm, Herbert and Ursula Koepf, following earlier meetings, visited the college and Francis invited Herbert to start a Biodynamic Agriculture Course at the college. They arrived in April 1970. Herbert was already 56 years of age when he joined the college. He had been involved in anthroposophy and committed to biodynamic agriculture ever since leaving school. After the war he went back to Hohenheim University, the leading agriculture college in Germany to complete his agricultural studies. He obtained his doctorate and continued as a Professor. He was there for 21 years. In 1961 he went to America where he worked with the American Biodynamic Association for four years before again returning to Hohenheim. As well as being an expert widely experienced in biodynamic agriculture he was a deeply read and serious anthroposophist, but without any dogma or fanaticism. He brought to the college an earnestness together with a sense of humour and a twinkle in his eye.

The Agriculture Course was launched properly in September 1971.

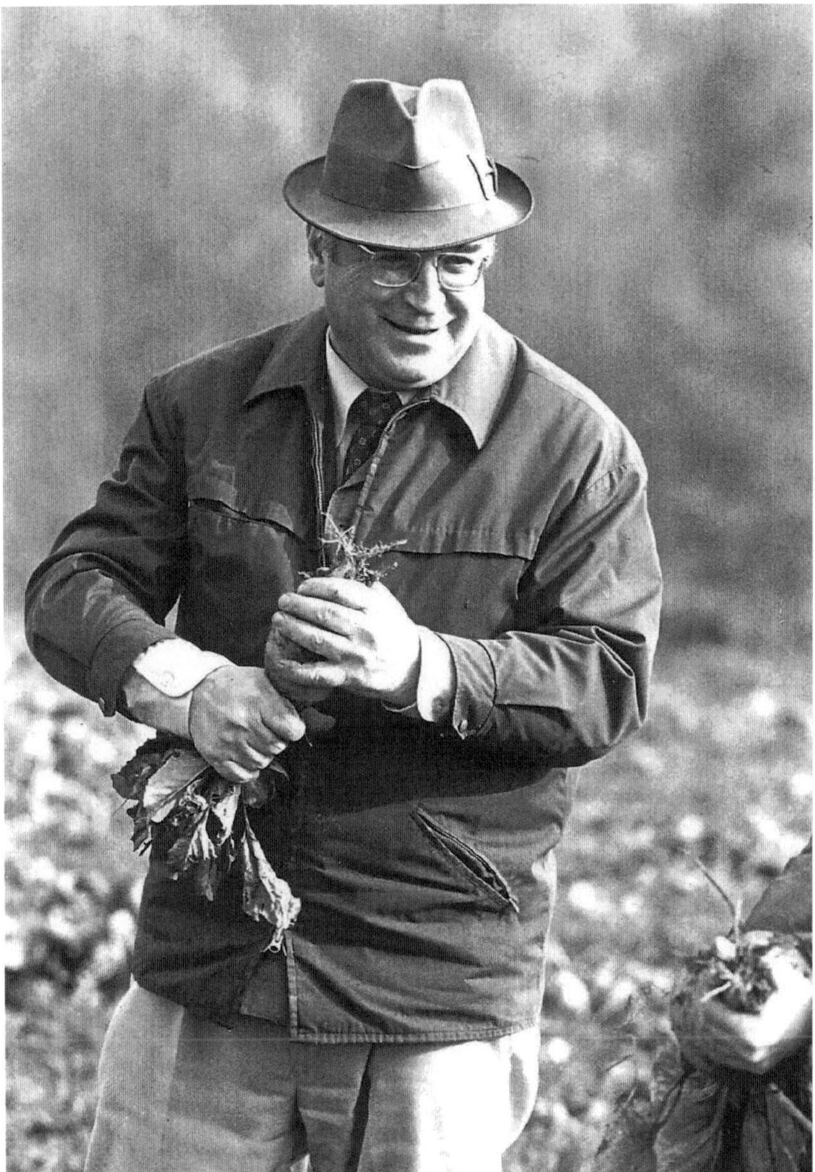

Herbert Koepf

The best I can do to describe it is to quote a passage from a paper Herbert later wrote:

> *Over the years the number of countries from which students came to the biodynamic training grew to just under 40. Some could afford to first take the Foundation Year, which proved to be very helpful for their further studies, but the majority could not. The very lively cultural and social life in the College compensated to some extend for the loss.*
>
> *Students were requested to have completed at least a year of hands-on training prior to joining. In fact the spectrum of those who arrived extended from having finished or interrupted a degree course, to just having practical experience. Hence in the first of the three terms an introduction to anthroposophy and some agriculture-related sciences was offered. Then followed climate, soils and conservation; biodynamic aspects of plant and animal husbandry; social economic aspects; quality of produce and consumer relations. Subsidiary topics such as gardening, fruit growing and agriculture in warm climates, were offered by guest lecturers. Field trips and occasional individual projects filled the programme.*
>
> *Central to the teaching process was an intensive group study, 110 sessions during two terms, of Rudolf Steiner's Agriculture Course which offers plenty of starting points to shed light on practical questions. Hands-on work included making and applying biodynamic preparations, composting, special seasonal jobs.*
>
> *This sounds like a greatly overcrowded programme. However it was not intended to cover all the details which could easily be obtained elsewhere or taken from a good textbook. It was the objective of this diverse curriculum to give an introduction to the many subjects from a biodynamic point of view; how to form environmentally orientated judgements and to kindle motivation. Some arts were offered throughout the year. All told, the group faced in the course of the year 12–15 teachers: farm and garden staff and guest lecturers.*
>
> *There was never any special advertising for the school, but every year the Course was full to a capacity which still allowed for individual attention, i.e. 15–25 students. Some of them are now in leading positions round the world.*

Though it was the intention that all students going into a training course would first complete the Foundation Year or its equivalent as he mentions above, it was not always practically or financially possible. Herbert particularly felt that for farmers there were many reasons why this might be impossible and also not always so necessary.

Herbert soon became involved in all agricultural and horticultural aspects of the work of the college both on the farm and the campus. In addition to the farm some students had started vegetable gardens on the college campus to provide fresh produce for the kitchen. To develop these more fully on an ongoing basis Herbert invited Annemarie Vinkhuyzen from Holland. She joined the college in October 1972. Her gardens were much frequented by both agriculture and other students. Some Foundation Year students also worked for certain periods with her as a craft element of their Course. Students often spoke of how working with Annemarie and her understanding of plants was a particularly valuable experience for them. In addition to the formal Course, a work-experience/apprentice programme was instituted both on Tablehurst Farm and with Annemarie in the garden. This developed over the years; they learnt mainly through the practical work on the farm or garden but also through classes arranged for them. They received board and lodging and pocket money. They usually stayed for one year, including summer, but some for two.

Herbert also instituted a certain amount of research within the Agriculture Course. For this he established a small research laboratory. Walter Goldstein who started as a student worked to develop this for some time before returning to America where he continued to develop his work in crop and soil research in the Michael Fields Agricultural Institute in Wisconsin. On the farm Herbert played an important part in the management of the farm and in a guiding and consultancy role. He regularly met with the farmers, more particularly so after Katherine Castelliz and Jeremy Kent had left.

Both Herbert and Ursula played important parts, beyond their teaching work, in the life of the college until they finally retired in 1991 when he was in his mid 70s. They then went for a few years to America before finally settling back in Germany.

The Rural Development Course (RDP)

Herbert Koepf met Mark and Chela Feedman in California in 1974–5. Following this meeting Mark and Chela came to study in the Agriculture Course in 1978–9. Mark had come with a deep impulse in his soul to develop a biodynamic agriculture programme appropriate to under-privileged people in underdeveloped countries. Even while he was a student he began planning to establish such a Course at Emerson. He would not take no for an answer. Many felt that this wealthy part of England was not the right place to start training people to work in countries with very different climate, social conditions, and soil fertility. However Mark was a man with a strong and determined will and great enthusiasm. On the Agriculture Course with him was Charles Griffin who was also interested. Mark recruited Charles to join him and in September 1979 the Course started with five students. Mark was also very active in travelling, particularly through Europe, working up support for his Course and raising much needed financial support. The Course was allocated a part of Parklands, the field just to the south of Pixton on the other side of the ha-ha. One thing I always remember about Mark, and something others have also commented on, was the importance of beauty and order in his gardens. Even the compost heaps had to be neat, in orderly rows, and well signed with details of when they were laid down. To him what a thing looked like was part of what it was.

During the following years student numbers fluctuated but generally increased to around 15 each year. The Course attracted some students from backgrounds very different from the normal at Emerson. This added a richness to the social life of the college. It directly added greatly to our awareness of the problems of people in the underdeveloped countries as well as highlighting questions of the place of modern technologies.

Matthias Guepin joined the staff in 1981. After many years biodynamic agricultural experience in Holland he took charge of the programme at Emerson and so left Mark free to develop a field station in the Dominican Republic. Mark became wholly involved there during 1982. The field station was developed as an independent enterprise separate from Emerson College itself. At the conference of anthroposophical banks in Driebergen, Holland, in February 1982 the banks pledged to support this work. They agreed to try to find an initial total of $45,000.

Hans Kern had been a student on the Agriculture Course and then on the RDP Course. In October 1982 he joined the staff of the Course. In 1985 Tadeo Caldas who had been a student in the Course the previous year joined the staff. Shortly after this Matthias went to Kenya to develop the work there. Tadeo then took charge of the Course. Irmfried Neuman also helped for a short period.

Sculpture Course

John Wilkes studied at the Royal College of Art in London. During that time he met George Adams who introduced him to projective—and what was then known as synthetic—geometry. He later worked as George's assistant in the Institute for Flow Sciences in Herrischried—

founded by George Adams and Theodor Schwenk. Later he also started working on the restoration of Rudolf Steiner's original plasticine models at the Goetheanum in Dornach.

In 1965 John was invited by Francis to develop sculptural activities at the college. He was at that time still working in Dornach. He could not leave this work immediately so to start with he came as a visiting teacher. This was while the college was still in the Huts. In 1968, just after the college moved to Pixton, he and his wife Alfhild moved into the top flat of Pixton House. He had still to complete his work in Dornach which he continued to do mainly in the holidays. It was not until November 1969 that he was able finally to commit himself fully to Emerson. From the beginning John taught sculpture in both the Foundation and Education Courses. In 1968–9 he also had a few students studying sculpture full-time with him. In 1971, in addition to his teaching-blocks to other Courses he started a full-time Sculpture Course with six students. This was a one-year Course and until the early 1980s the numbers remained comparatively small.

In addition to his teaching John continued his research work into the movement and flow of water. He was given space in the attic of the new barn on the farm for this purpose. Rudolf Kaesbach, who had earlier been a student in John's Course, had came back in July 1981 to assist in the

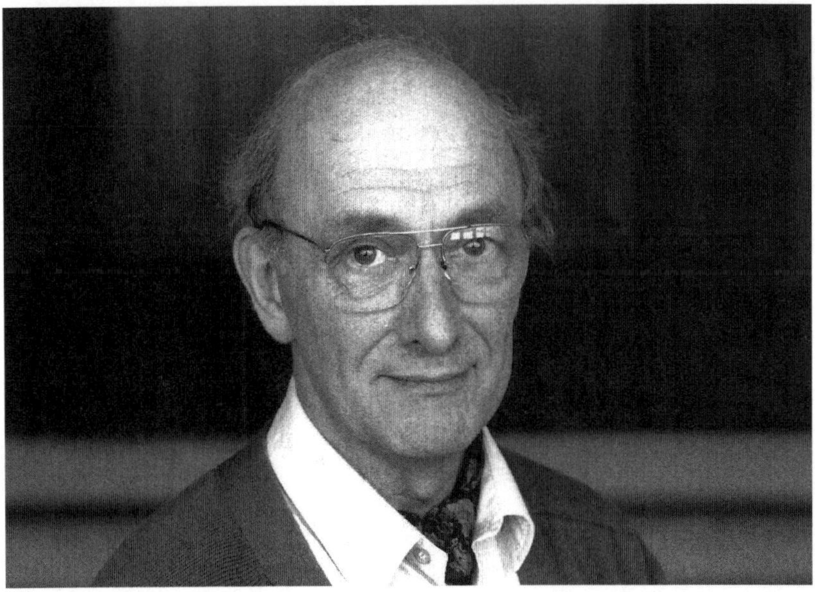

John Wilkes

Sculpture Course. This made it possible for John to give more time to his research work and to the development of Flowforms. Over the next few years Rudolf increasingly took over the actual teaching and the running of the Course. He extended the full-time Course to three years and student numbers slowly increased into the 20s.

Flow Research

Adult education and training is always invigorated when accompanied by research. When Francis invited John Wilkes to teach sculpture at the college he was prompted to do so also by the research John was working on. He saw the importance of this area of work and he wanted to support it. John had become particularly interested in water and its movement. At an early time in his research he came to the observation and question: in all living organisms there is symmetry but, except in the crystal, there is no symmetry in the world of matter—in the mineral. What happens if we offer symmetry to water? This question led to the development of Flowforms.

An indication of his work can be seen in a paragraph in the Forward to his book *Flowforms**:

> *Such surfaces, as Adams discovered—and presented in his book with Olive Whicher,* The Plant Between Sun and Earth—*are fundamental to the forms of living organisms. Thus water and its relationship to these special mathematically describable surfaces was to be investigated with regard to possible influences on the water. Water and surface are inseparable. Water is always moving over surfaces and, over shorter or longer periods, depending on the erodible nature of the material, the shape of those surfaces is influenced. Water in movement always tends to create a multitude of surfaces within itself but these can be influenced by the condition of the water. In a living context water movement plays a major creative role in formative processes. Indeed every physical forming process is at some time in a fluid state.*

Many people became interested in, and sensed the importance of, John's work. Some, after studying with him at Emerson, helped take it out into the world—people such as Nigel Wells, Andrew Joiner, Herbert Dreiseitl, Iain Trousdell, and others.

Nick Weidmann came as a student to the Foundation Year in 1983. He then joined the Sculpture Course. In 1987 he joined the staff to work

* Floris Books 2003.

with John Wilkes and has continued to the present time doing much of the practical aspects of the research, as well as occasionally teaching.

The story of the development of the Flowforms, of the setting up of the Flowform Design Company Ltd and of the growth to a worldwide activity is beyond the scope of this book. But it was an important and ongoing piece of research and development, inspired by John Wilkes, that was given a place at Emerson and which in turn enriched the life of the college. It showed what can be developed when science and art are brought together.

The Christian Community Priest Training

This started in 1969. Although it was included in the wider umbrella of Emerson College, it was actually run separately at Shalesbrooke by priests of the Christian Community. The students did join the Foundation Year for some studies. There was also an important connection through their housing some of our students in Shalesbrooke. Adam Bittleston also had weekly open discussion evenings to which some of our students went and found very helpful. The Course closed in the mid-'70s when, I believe, it moved to Germany.

Painting Course

Francis Edmunds had met and come to know Anne Stockton during his visits to America. She was then in her mid-50s, a long-standing anthroposophist and a painting teacher in the New York Waldorf School. He recognized her deep commitment to anthroposophy and was interested in her work and her impulses in the realm of colour. He invited her to come to Emerson to teach painting. She joined the college in July 1968. Being American, what she brought in her own being of that country was a great addition to the staff of the college, particularly as so many of our students came from that continent. Many students also valued her deep studies in anthroposophy and her experience in working with what she had come to understand of it.

In 1970 Anne also started a Painting Course with five students. The space and facilities at the college did not allow her to develop this in the way she felt necessary so in 1979 she left the college to found her own school of painting which she named Tobias School of Art. At first this found a home in Bank Cottage Farm on the edge of the golf course in Forest Row. Later it acquired a new and permanent home in Peredur at East Grinstead where it continued to develop successfully. Her son,

Manning Goodwin, whom I have already mentioned on several occasions, supported her in this initiative.

Independent Programmes

Most years there were some students who, having attended the Foundation Year and not being attracted to one of the training courses, wished to stay on to work further with a particular teacher or to work more extensively in a particular craft or art for which there was no regular Course. Consideration was always given to such requests. Provided the teacher concerned had time and agreed and the facilities were available without impinging on the regular Courses, individual arrangements would be agreed. Most years there were some students on such arrangements.

Eurythmy

A group of Foundation Year students whose destiny had brought them together, mostly in the Foundation Year of 1972–3, requested the college to start a eurythmy training course for them. They had all met eurythmy working with Elizabeth Edmunds and resolved to take it up as their life's work. They were a serious and committed group of young people and this was obviously a serious request, so it was given earnest consideration by the college, particularly by Elizabeth, Francis, John Davy and me. There were, of course, many problems to be overcome. A proper eurythmy training would last a minimum of four years. The college could not commit itself to such a long training. So if there was to be a shorter start to a training it would have to be done in conjunction with a fully established existing training school who would be prepared to oversee it and accept the students into its own Course at the end of the one or two years at Emerson. The person we found to run it would have to be someone they had confidence in and with whom they could work.

There were at that time tentative plans to move the London School of Eurythmy to East Grinstead. The college recognized the necessity of their not feeling this new Course as a threat to their own work and that they supported the new initiative. The college would also have to obtain the support of the Eurythmy section in Dornach. After a number of lengthy discussions between the college and Marguerite Lundgren and Cecil Harwood of the London School of Eurythmy, and Dr. Hagen Biesantz of Dornach, it was eventually agreed that the Course would go ahead. Molly von Heider was invited to take responsibility for the training. She was a eurythmist of many years' experience both in training eurythmists and in teaching children in Waldorf Schools. She was also a person of considerable life experience and wisdom. Roger Yates who already taught eurythmy at the college would work with her. Marguerite Lundgren would have some involvement in the Course, including some teaching.

The Course started in September 1973 with 12 students and ran for two years. Else Klink of the Stuttgart School of Eurythmy in Germany recognized the value of this work and most of the students went on to complete their training with her. The Course was popular but experience showed that it was better for students to transfer into a full training after one year rather than two, so subsequent courses were all for one year only. Course numbers increased to 20 by 1979–80 and then declined. In 1981–2, for a number of reasons, it was decided to discontinue the Course. Molly had passed retirement age but still wanted to start a one-term Course for preparing trained eurythmists to teach children.

Education Eurythmy

Molly started this Course, for those who intended to teach eurythmy to children, in September 1982 with 11 students from various eurythmy schools. Again this Course was very successful and ran for some eight years. Helen Bawden later joined Molly and eventually took over from her. At that time there was a certain friction between the various eurythmy schools. With students from different schools Molly was able to work in a way that the differences in their trainings brought depth to their performances rather than division. I remember also the joy in their playing when Molly was able to get them to behave as though they were again small children.

Cooking

By the year 1974–5 Anthony Kaye and his helpers in the kitchen were cooking for around 180 students and staff, three meals a day, seven days a week. This was a time when there was still little consciousness in the wider society of the importance of a healthy diet. Due to Anthony's cooking Emerson food had acquired a widespread reputation and a number of aspiring young cooks wanted to learn from him. He therefore started a Cooking Course. This was more in the nature of an apprenticeship rather than a full-time Course. But there were between three and five students who joined the college to work with him on this basis for the next four years, that is, until Anthony left the college to go back to farming.

The Social Development Centre

This was founded in 1975 by Coen van Houten and Christopher Schaefer. Coen and Christopher had both worked for some years at the Netherlands Pedagogical Institute (NPI) in Holland founded by Dr Bernard Lievegoed. The work of the Centre was to a large extent founded on the work of that Institute, but Coen and Christopher very much wanted it to be within Emerson College. It was not possible at that time to house the new impulse within the existing college buildings; they were already very overcrowded. Nor had the college the financial resources to acquire a new property. If the new Centre was to come into being under the overall umbrella of Emerson College it would have to find its own buildings and necessary capital. This, after much effort and with considerable support from friends, it succeeded in doing.

On 26 September 1975 the Centre opened with the first Course of 17 students in Bjerkley, a house lent as a temporary home by Manning Goodwin. During 1976 Old Plaw Hatch House was purchased and in September of that year the Centre moved into its future home, now with 22 students. Old Plaw Hatch House is in Sharpthorne, about five miles from Pixton. Legally the Centre was part of the college; the Council of Management carried overall responsibility for its activities, its students were registered as students of Emerson College. But it also had considerable independence. There was much about it that came out of Bernard Lievegoed's NPI rather than that of Francis Edmunds's impulse behind Emerson College. I often sensed that Francis was not always comfortable about this difference. The welcoming of this impulse into the college came much more from John Davy than from Francis.

They organized and ran their own Courses, found their own staff and teachers and made their own social arrangements within the Centre. They also ran their own accounts, had their own bank account and paid their own bills. But salaries and taxes, etc. were calculated and paid as part of the whole by Jean and myself in Pixton. The accounts of the Centre were audited and incorporated into the main college accounts at the end of each year. Their earlier teachers still did a considerable amount of private consultancy work within the wider world of business and industry, from which work they drew much of their income. This direct contact with organizations active in the wider world, both large and small, was important and greatly strengthened their work as well as relieving pressure on the cost of salaries. Over the years they had some interesting people join their staff, who also contributed to the life of the college as a whole.

These included Djobs van Houten, Tijno Voors, Steve Briault, and later Ernst Amons and Clara Passchier.

There was always at least one member of the staff of the Centre on the Council of Management as well as some sharing of teachers. For a number of years, until they established their own cooking arrangements, they drew their main meal each day from the college kitchens at Pixton. Due to the distance between the Centre and the main college campus the two tended to have their own distinct and individual social lives. But some students from Pixton did go to the weekly evening lectures and to certain other events. Centre students and staff also often came to the festivals and other social events at Pixton.

It is not my intention to go further in this book into the life and work of the Social Development Centre. Here my intention is to look, as far as I am able, at all that arose directly out of the impulse of Francis Edmunds in founding the college. The story of the Social Development Centre really needs to be written as something standing in its own right. But I should say that, whatever the differences in the impulses at work in each, many of their staff made important contributions to the life of the college. Like in the college itself, towards the end of the 1980s student numbers began to dwindle and eventually, in the early 1990s, the Centre had to close.

Voice Training Course

Ursula Koepf came to the college in 1970 when her husband Herbert Koepf was invited to start the Agriculture Course. Like him she brought with her a long and deep commitment to anthroposophy. In her biographical notes she admits to being reluctant to move to England from her home in Germany. But she then states:

> *And then the 'College'! We entered in a life, which was—to say the least—unusual! There was a structure but nevertheless it was left to the teachers in a very free way to develop their courses, their teaching. There was a group of 'pioneers', experts in their fields, deeply rooted in Anthroposophy and its practical application to serve the questions and searching of the students. Students not in the normal sense but people from all walks of life who often after years of professional work began to question the deeper sense of it and what their true destiny is.*

Ursula had trained in, and had also been teaching, singing. At Emerson she soon entered fully into the community life and brought to it her particular gifts. She regularly invited musicians from outside to give concerts at the college and so added an important musical richness, not only to the college but to the area. She began working with individual students teaching them singing. In September 1982 she developed this into a Voice Course with six students. By 1986–7 student numbers had increased to 14.

Speech & Drama

In 1983–4 an Intermediate or Middle Year was started. This was for students who had completed the Foundation Year but felt they needed a year of arts and crafts before going into a full training. The following year 1984–5 there were insufficient students for it except for a group of 11 wanting to work at speech and drama with Dawn Langman. From this the Speech and Drama Course started, later led by Sarah Kane. Ashley Ramsden joined the college in 1988 to help with this Course. Later, during the '90s, he initiated the Story-Telling Courses.

Witten Annen English Language Course

In 1981 we were approached by the Witten Annen teacher-training college in Germany. They had students who intended to teach English in German Waldorf schools so needed to prepare for and take the Cambridge Proficiency in English Examination. Could this be done at Emerson? The proposal was that Witten Annen would pay us a lump sum annually and we would organize the Course at Emerson to which they would send not more than 10 students each year. Students would pay their own board and lodging but no tuition fee which would be covered by the lump sum payment. The Course would be run within the Foundation Year framework—it would run in the mornings and the students would participate in the Foundation Year art and craftwork in the afternoons.

The college agreed to this and took on Ann Horscroft, an experienced and qualified teacher to run it. The Course started in September 1981. Eginhard Fuchs, one of the founding teachers of Witten Annen was our contact and he became a regular visitor and friend of the college. In fact regular contacts developed between the two colleges. An interesting detail was that when their teachers visited and talked to our teachers about the students there was at the beginning confusion as to whom they were talking about. They knew their students by their family names, whereas our teachers knew them just by their given or first names.

Ann was a good teacher and the students did well, but there was always the problem that she had no connection to, or interest in, anthroposophy. It was the first time the college had employed someone in this way. It did not in itself create any problems but it was strange to have someone in the community who played no part in it, who just came, did her work, and left to her own other world. Later the college arranged for Andrew Wolpert to take over the course. He was a man who had worked with anthroposophy for many years and was also a qualified and experienced teacher of the English language to foreigners. His own command of the English language made him a joy to listen to.

10
The Arts and Crafts

In addition to the Courses described in the last two chapters there were a number of art and craft activities that contributed to the Courses and which for a few students were a source of special studies, or of quiet therapeutic activity in the evenings and at weekends.

Just as there could often be sensed permeating the social life of the college something of the discussions, questions, and inner challenges students were working with in their Courses, so there was also an ever present sense of artistic and craft creative activity. The joy of discovering the creativity within oneself could often be sensed, for example at meal times when they talked of what they had just been working on. It was surprising how many students had never actually done anything in the way of artistic or craft activity before coming to the college. They now discovered that it is possible for anyone to create, to bring an inner truth or feeling to expression in artistic form, or make something that is both functional and beautiful. The sense of achievement can be enormously encouraging and confidence-building to a young person who had previously too often been led to believe he had no such talents. Somehow any sense of competition never arose amongst the students; it did not matter if one was still at the beginning while others were more advanced. It was just a matter of each person being at a different point on their journey of self-discovery. Everyone could participate in the joy and excitement that a person experienced, particularly one who had never had an opportunity to be creative before. This often came to expression in the House Meetings and in the presentations of student work.

Not all the arts and crafts were running at the same time. There were also the Christmas plays and the end of year play, usually a Shakespeare. I describe these more fully in chapter 12.

Eurythmy

In eurythmy students could experience the sounds expressed in speech and music, as movement. This was something that students from all Courses did for some period of their time at the college. Although there were always some people (usually men) who did not like it, most were deeply appreciative, particularly of Elizabeth Edmunds as a teacher. Through her a number went on to a full training. It was taught and led by Elizabeth from the beginning. She was later joined by a number of other teachers including Valery Soukup, Alfhild Wilkes, Roger Yates, Doris Meeks, Melissa Stone (Harwood) Glenys Waters, and Christopher Kidman. As the number of Courses increased it became quite a juggling exercise to arrange for a teacher and a suitable space for each, especially as most Courses preferred the coffee to lunch period for such activities.

Sculpture

Sculpture was described more fully in the last chapter. This was an artistic activity in which students explore the qualities of form more intensively. It was included within different Courses and as a full-time Course in itself. Like painting, sculpture was considered one of the basic artistic activities that every student should experience. John Wilkes started teaching while the college was still in the Huts. Rudolf Kaesbach, a former student who joined the staff in 1981 later took responsibility for this work.

Painting

As mentioned earlier, from 1968 Anne Stockton taught painting, particularly as an exploration of colour, in the various courses. This was also considered to be one of the more important artistic activities that every student should participate in.

Speech and Drama

Mechthild Harkness taught speech and drama, with particular focus on the relationship between word and gesture, in 1967–8. After Mechthild left Graham Rickett took over. He taught speech within the Courses and helped with the drama work which was mainly carried by Francis Edmunds. Later Grahame Hope carried the speech teaching.

Weaving, Spinning and Dyeing

Weaving, spinning and dyeing are prime examples of practical exercises in the training of thought. This was a very popular series of crafts and most evenings there were students working at their looms. Dana Prager was invited to join the college in 1968 to teach them, which she did with great success, much appreciated by those who chose to work with her. Rachel Horsfall assisted her for many years.

Woodcraft

In 1968 Francis Edmunds invited Peter Horsfall to join the college in order to teach woodcarving. This included an exploration of the nature of woods from different trees and their qualities. Like many of the craft teachers Peter brought a moral quality of life to his craft and students greatly valued this.

Singing—Choir & Orchestra

Francis often spoke of the importance of singing as a community activity for the whole college. Julian Pook, previously a student, joined as a staff member in 1971 and organized and taught both a choir and, when there were enough instrumentalists, an orchestra. Many Courses liked to have some singing, either to start the day or as an artistic activity. As mentioned above, Ursula Koepf also taught singing and took over the choir when Julian left in 1983.

Poetry and Creative Writing

Paul Matthews, another former student, joined the staff part-time in 1972 on a sort of apprenticeship while teaching at Michael Hall, and then

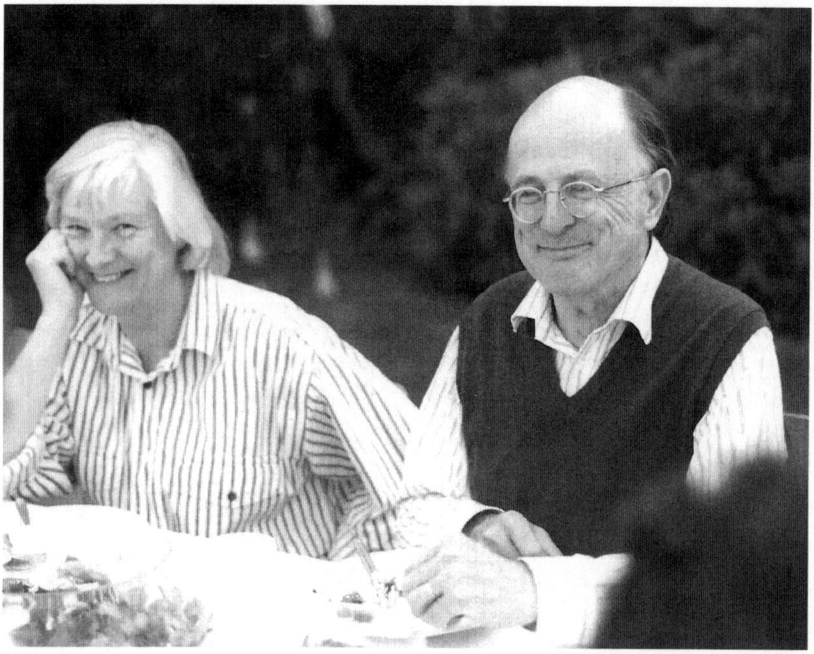

Rachel and Peter Horsfall

became full-time in 1980. Amongst other activities he taught poetry and later creative writing as a training of the imagination through the art of word.

Bothmer Gymnastics
Bothmer gymnastics involved developing rhythmical movements of the limbs within space. With Olive Whicher, Paul Matthews taught gymnastics to those who asked for it. This was usually an extracurricula activity in the early mornings. From 1974 to 1976 there was an actual training course, partly at Emerson and partly at Michael Hall.

Pottery
This is very much a craft of creating through the activity and sensitivity of the hands. Ann Druitt (then Ann Borries) joined the college in 1968 as part-student and part-teacher to start the pottery. She established this in what had been the dog-kennels and carried it for three years. When she left there was no one to follow her so it became a sort of periodic craft.

Glove Puppets
With glove puppets students learnt to bring new and expressive movements through their hands. Gisela Bittleston for many years taught puppetry to a few students in her caravan. She had a very particular style and students intending to work with small children were particularly drawn to her.

Bookbinding
Lionel Elin taught bookbinding, a craft that demands exceptional precision. Because of the nature of his arthritic body he was not able to teach more than three or four at a time, but despite this handicap he was extremely skilled and did beautiful work. Many of the students he did work with spoke of the ability he had to teach a morality of truthfulness through the craft—truth and honesty had to inform every aspect of it. For many it was an important experience to work with such a man who suffered in the way he did and yet carried out such skilled work without ever complaining. Conrad Saxon-Snell, who had worked closely with him, took over in the late 1970s. I can find no record of exactly when.

Gardening
Gardening, the only outdoor craft, was included in the Foundation Year Course. There were some students who very much valued working with

Annemarie Vinkhuyzen and learning so much about plants and nature in the actual doing of the work of the garden. It was also a strong balancing contrast to much of the intense head-work of the Course.

Batik

Out of her working with costumes Roswitha Spence developed her work with batik. She began teaching this as an afternoon activity in the Foundation Year. Batik, the dyeing of fabric using hot wax to create design, is an activity that calls for both craftsmanship as well as artistic creativity. Roswitha was someone able to work creatively in both these disciplines.

Form Drawing

Alongside batik Roswitha began teaching form drawing, the art of line, in the Foundation Year as a morning activity. She was also asked to teach this in several other courses in blocks. It was the way she brought her anthroposophical understanding into her classes that attracted many students.

Puppetry

Francis Edmunds and John Davy both encouraged Roswitha to take up puppetry as an exploration of the human form and its expression in movement. She resisted this for some years but eventually in the mid-1980s began developing it, again as a Foundation Year afternoon Course. This work developed considerably over the following years.

Handcrafts

Gerda Hillman, who had been a regular visiting teacher, was invited to join the college full-time in 1974 to teach handwork, the making of soft toys and dolls, to the aspiring teachers in the Education Course. She was then in her late 60s. She had been a pupil in the first Waldorf School in Stuttgart and so had known Rudolf Steiner through personal experience. She brought special qualities from this, and many delightful stories. Her love of children and years of experience working with them and her sense of humour added a richness to her classes.

11
The Non-Teaching Activities

In chapter 7 I spoke about Margaret Fox and of her work as falling within the economic sphere of activity. It is seldom clear whether a particular activity rightly belongs in one or other of the three spheres of social life—it practically never falls wholly but only mainly in one. This is not the place to go into this question. Nevertheless, it can be helpful to look at it as follows:

Teaching, the basic purpose of the college, is clearly an activity of the cultural life of the community. Both the teacher and the student find, in the first place, the purpose and meaning of their working together within the depths of their own souls. It is a fulfilling of their own soul impulses.

It is quite different for those working on the more practical needs of the college, the non-teaching activities. While some non-teacher activities such as cooking or gardening can be partially fulfilling in themselves, the work in the office doing the accounts on a computer, keeping the floors and toilets clean and healthy or maintaining the buildings and equipment, are requirements arising out of the practical life of the community, not out of a person's own soul needs. It is not possible to find the same meaning and purpose in this work as in, for example, teaching. Such work generally has no purpose in itself; it is done in order to make possible the work between teacher and student. The non-teaching activities in the college broadly, though not entirely, come into the economic sphere of activity. In nearly every way the nature of economic work is opposite to cultural activity.

When categorizing people working in an organization such as Emerson College into 'teachers' and 'non-teaching staff' there is always a tendency to do this in a way that brings division between the two groups. In some anthroposophical organizations this division has even gone so far as to assume that anthroposophists should be involved in more creative activity. Those in the office are sometimes seen as employed to do certain work, it not being necessary for them to be interested in or to understand the anthroposophical work of the organization.

* * *

At Emerson we tried to keep conscious of the fact that we were all, in our different tasks, carriers of the work of the college; we were colleagues and as such each was important within the whole. The non-teachers made possible the work of the teachers, whose work in turn gave meaning and purpose to the work of the non-teachers. I have already mentioned elsewhere something of this and of the particular importance of the Staff Meeting. From the beginning and up to quite late in the life of the college, the great majority, if not all, of those who joined to carry the non-teaching work came out of their own initiatives or through personal connections—brought to the college by their destinies. The college soon became a community of work which people wanted to join, not so much for the particular work itself, but to be part of the wider impulse of the college. We never formally advertised in the normal way when we needed someone, whether to teach or for the work in the office, kitchen, maintenance or elsewhere; we either approached a particular person we knew or who had already expressed interest, or we spread word of our need to other related organizations.

Within the staff there was generally a strong commitment to the work of the college as a whole and a real interest in the students. This love for, and interest in, the whole was sometimes stronger in the non-teachers than in the teachers who, of necessity, were more focused on their particular students and work. There was not a clear divide between teachers and non-teachers. Many teachers took on or helped with non-teaching work and some staff whose main responsibilities lay in the non-teaching areas of work also did some teaching. It was also recognized that all non-teaching staff in their different ways, at some time, came into contact with, and in many situations actually worked with, students. For some students their involvement with non-teachers, who were also in their different ways working with anthroposophy, was often an important part of their experience and of their meeting anthroposophy in the everyday tasks of life. Students found that they could sometimes talk to a non-teacher on a level they could not do with a teacher. Non-teachers often met aspects of students, or sensed problems that were hidden from the teacher.

The recognition of all staff being co-carriers of the work, of being colleagues in one work, was consciously maintained. Not only was it important for the staff themselves, but it was part of the overall experience of the students, and therefore of the educational element they gained from the college.

⋆ ⋆ ⋆

It is not possible to say something about each of the many people who have helped over the years in the various non-teaching areas of the college, many of whom came for only a short time, or were really students working their way through. But I shall try to say something, even if no more than their name, about all those who made a more ongoing contribution to the life and work of the college. It is important to remember that Emerson arose out of the vision and intuition of one man, Francis Edmunds. He gathered together the people who would develop and carry it forward. It was part of his genius to then leave it to the many people who came to contribute in so many ways to form it and to fulfil the task for which he had brought it into being. Everyone who worked at the college, in whatever capacity, was involved somehow in that work.

When I joined the college in the last year in the Huts, Lionel Elin looked after the accounts and Margaret Fox was secretary to Francis Edmunds. In the kitchen Anthony Kaye with his assistant Gwyneth Sutherland and with assistance from students, produced all the meals. Marcia Elin ran a small bookstall and Jeremy Kent looked after the gardens while doing some teaching. Apart from Gwyneth I have already said something about these people who continued after the move to Pixton.

The Offices

Up to around the middle of the 1970s all correspondence with students applying to attend the college, and acceptances of their applications, was dealt with by Francis. John Davy then began to take over from him. It was recognized that in this work one was dealing with people's destinies and with the intentions and impulses they brought with them through birth. It was a matter of course that acceptance of a student could not be based merely on their meeting certain requirements of age, experience, and ability to pay, but on deeper considerations that needed to be dealt with by someone who had prepared himself through anthroposophical studies and an ongoing work on a meditative path of inner development. Later, as the training courses grew the Course leaders took over much of this work.

Margaret Fox continued to work part-time for Francis Edmunds looking after all his correspondence and maintaining the filing system. She later worked also for John Davy as he took over much of what Francis had been carrying. She retired in 1980 when, if I remember rightly, she reached 60 years of age. Both she and her husband, David, had only learned to drive since they were 50. They had bought a small car and now enjoyed exploring the countryside and trips down to the coast.

After Margaret left Jo Iliffe joined the staff to take over her work. She stayed for four years and in 1984 Sonia Argy was invited to continue the work, now almost entirely with John Davy.

By early 1970, with 85 full-time students and increasing numbers of staff, coping with all the accounts for the expanding college and the developing farm was getting too much for me on top of all the other work I was doing. So it was agreed I should have an assistant. We heard that Jean Pryor (later Jean Steele), who had been in the same class as myself at Michael Hall School, was out of work and looking for something. Roswitha phoned her. She had just started a new job but after some persuasion from Roswitha agreed to come down to help out for two weeks. She came but never went back. Jean worked with me keeping the accounts for the next 21 years. During this time she met John Steele who was then working at Plaw Hatch Farm. Their wedding was a college social occasion. In 1991 she retired to spend more time with John, who was considerably older than her. When he died a few years later she returned to continue part-time looking after the accounts. As I write she is still there and, like the Queen and her Prime Ministers, has seen through quite a number of bursars, and financial directors.

Jean and I worked closely together. We each brought different capacities to the work and so made a good team. Neither of us had had any training in accountancy so we had to sort out new problems in accounting as they arose. The auditors were always impressed and said they found it difficult to believe that we had had no training. She was, and still is, totally committed to the college. Of course in the early days there were no computers so it was all book entry. Then later we had to master computer accountancy. I was interested but also concerned that in working with computers I lost a certain sensing of the flow of the money, a feeling of how the college was doing each year. Between us we kept all the accounts for the college as well as for the farm. This included paying salaries, issuing bills to the students and collecting their payments, as well as chasing up the slow payers. We paid all bills, including calculating and paying rents to the landladies. We also, as mentioned earlier, ran a sort of banking service for students after lunch when they could cash cheques, change foreign money or draw money from their account. I say 'we' but most of this work fell on Jean as I was also involved in other work.

Ann Gooding joined the office in 1976. She became a sort of receptionist as well as doing much of the typing of letters, notices, and papers for any members of staff who needed something done that they could not do themselves. She also compiled and produced the weekly bulletin which went to all Courses and the noticeboard. Before computers we had a Gestetner for printing quantities of circulars or other documents. This was a messy business inevitably ending with inky fingers. But she seemed to master it. Ann had a great sense of humour, particularly of the ways of the upper-classes from which she herself had come. When invited to she declined joining the Emerson Association as she said she was not really an anthroposophist. But she was deeply connected to the college and later when the financial situation got difficult she decided she did not need a salary on top of her own income.

As the college continued to expand and the demands on the office grew accordingly a number of other people were taken on periodically to help in the office, mostly students working their way through one or other Course.

Student Housing

Roswitha carried this work for the first seven years after the move to Pixton. By the year 1973–4 student numbers had reached around 150. We still had only the 16 purpose-built rooms on campus plus Shalesbrooke and some other housing in the village, so the great majority of students still needed to be housed, and rooms for these had to be found with landladies in the village. In addition there were now sometimes up to six or seven families coming from abroad who needed a house. This was an enormous task. In 1974 the responsibility for student housing was passed to Myra Macdonald, assisted by her husband Alistair Macdonald. Student numbers continued to increase over the next few years and in the early 1980s the summer Courses and conferences were developed. These also put great pressure on the Housing Team so in 1980 Rachel Horsfall joined them. This was only slightly eased in 1984 when Westwood student house with 24 rooms and a staff flat was opened.

Myra and Alistair were a special couple who contributed greatly to the life of the college and particularly to the welfare of the students. Alistair had been a barrister and was involved in or chaired a number of government enquiries. He was now retired. Their own children had all grown but they loved caring for young people. Alistair's first involvement in the college was running one of *The Philosophy of Freedom* study groups for the Foundation Year. They also often invited students to their home for tea and cakes. Many students have mentioned the importance of this. Like so many of the other older contributors this was all a gift, they never asked for any payment. Rachel Horsfall was a person who seemed to have no speciality but contributed in so many different ways. She never seemed to panic or get in a fluster. She could be a great calming influence. I have shown elsewhere how she ran the crèche for the young children so that the mothers could attend lectures. She also helped Dana teaching spinning, dyeing, and weaving and has over the years helped out when needed in the office. And later she helped in carrying the enormous task of housing the students.

The Kitchen

I have already written of Anthony Kaye and the place of the kitchen and the meals within the social life of the college (particularly in chapters 6 and 13). Gwyneth Sutherland, the sister of John Wilkes, who had also worked in the kitchen in the Huts came back to work with Anthony from 1968 to 1971. Two other local ladies I remember working with him during the early days in Pixton were Shirley Keymer and Angela Buckham. Marsalaidh Clark was another who worked in the kitchen from 1972 until 1975. She later came back to take over as Housemother.

Anthony was called back to Ireland in early 1978 to take over a family biodynamic farm. Two people, Martin Ekama and Wendy Cook, who had been working with him, were able to step in to take charge of the kitchen until another more experienced and permanent replacement could be found. Luckily Irene Bruntsch came forward to take over the kitchen. She came from Germany and joined in September 1978. Irene was also a very socially-minded person and in her own way continued to maintain much of the particular social orientation of the kitchen that Anthony had established. She also became active in the general life of the college.

There were, of course, many others who for longer or shorter periods worked in the kitchen. Some were part-time students working their way through the college, or working one year to help cover the fees the following year. Some had found their way to Emerson and just wanted, for a period, to be part of the community. Others, such as Wobbe van der Wegt, Hugh Ratcliffe, Heather Goodwin and Suzette Beadsmore (later Griffin), mostly former students, helped carry the kitchen over longer periods of time. Unfortunately there are no records now available of all the many others who helped carry this work over the years. We did not often have difficulty keeping the kitchen staffed with helpers. Sometimes it was difficult to convince a person that we could not take anyone else on, even for just board and lodging. The kitchen space was too small to have a large staff.

In 1987 Irene had to return to Germany and Franz Christen was taken on to head up the kitchen team. He brought considerable experience and an element of professionalism to the kitchen that it had not had before. His wife Katherine was a former student and had been one of those behind the request for the eurythmy training course. At its peak in the 1980s the kitchen was providing up to 250 lunches a day, as well as breakfasts and suppers and weekend meals. In addition to the college at Pixton (students and staff) it provided lunches for the Social Development Centre.

Housemother

Elizabeth Edmunds cared for the students and through her artistic and loving nature ensured Pixton became a homely and welcoming house. For the first few years at Pixton, she it was who guided a group of students who took responsibility for maintaining the house and organizing the cleaning.

Helen O'Reilly had been a Housemother and cook in Cotswold Chine in Gloucester. She came first as a Foundation Year student but stayed on as Housemother. She was a lively and efficient woman who helped to establish form in the house and in the cleaning organization. In 1973 she retired to join her family in Australia. Ilse Brice came to us to take over from Helen. She had been a Housemother in Potterspury Homes and had just retired, but wanted still to be active. She was a motherly woman who looked after the house and mothered the students for the next 12 years. She brought with her considerable experience of caring for people in anthroposophical homes. She strove to make the house a warm, homely and cheerful place for the students.

Then Marsalaidh Clark, who had also worked in the kitchen, came back to take over as Housemother in April 1985. The college had increased considerably in size and the work became too much for Ilse in her 70s. She stayed on in a small flat adapted for her on the campus, until she eventually had to move into a nursing home where she eventually died. Marsalaidh was able to bring considerable energy to organizing student work to cope with the expanded situation of the college. She had previously had nursing training and experience so was able to develop this aspect of the task of the Housemother.

Maintenance

As already mentioned, in 1968 John Bradley, a former student from the Huts was invited by Francis to create a workshop and to take responsibility for the repairs and maintenance at the college, and the farm machinery. He developed the workshop in one of the farm buildings. But he was not able to continue as hoped and left in 1970. He was followed by Hugh Taylor, Fred Dowle, Tom Birmingham, and John Nunnerly who in turn over the following 12 years carried this work to enable them, or their wives, to attend Courses.

In 1982 Andrew Joiner was invited to join as a full-time member of staff in order to bring more continuity to this work which had been expanding with the increase in buildings. Through working with John Wilkes he became interested in water and decided to take this further. He left in summer 1988.

Oliver Fynes-Clinton had been a member of the Pixton Builders. He joined the maintenance team with Andrew Joiner in September 1985 and took main responsibility for it when Andrew left. He was someone able to enter fully into the life of the college and enjoyed working with students. Christine, his wife, was also connected to the college as a visiting teacher for the Education Course and worked with Ann Druitt in running Lifeways—the summer Course.

Another person who contributed a great deal was Conrad Saxon-Snell. His main area of work could generally be included under maintenance. But he was one of those who wanted no money, but just to contribute in whatever way he could, to belong somewhere. He loved to help people. He started by helping John Wilkes cleaning the skeletons of dead animals for the sculpture department. John acquired the bodies of animals that had died from the zoo and these had to be stripped of their flesh to expose the beautiful forms of their bones. At one point, with his own money, he greatly improved the stage-lighting. Then later he took over the teaching of bookbinding from Lionel Elin.

Another person who was always ready to help, and did so particularly in the maintenance department was John Steele.

Garden

The vegetable garden to the north of Ruskin was started in 1971 by a student, Sherry Slotoroff, as a student project. She and others put a lot of work into getting this going. At that time there were neither hedges nor the line of trees beyond—it was an open wind-swept hillside. As I mentioned in chapter 9, in 1972 Annemarie Vinkhuyzen was invited by Herbert Koepf to take over and develop the vegetable garden and to work with students. She worked with the agriculture students and also with those Foundation Year students who chose it as a craft. She produced fresh vegetables for the kitchen which were much appreciated. Her real interest was working with vegetables but she also helped look after the lawns and flower gardens. The college had not been in a position to employ anyone specifically to care for these—the work had always been done by students as part of the domestic work arrangements. This continued, but now Annemarie brought overall planning and supervision to the work.

Annemarie, like Jean with her accounts, though almost 80 but still with considerable energy, continues to work in the garden, though no longer carrying responsibility for it. She has always joined fully in the social life, and has made sure that there were flowers for the festivals and other special occasions.

Library

From the beginning the college had begun to accumulate books for a library. In 1970 Barbara Saunders Davies stepped in to work three afternoons a week to care for it. She was then also in charge of the anthroposophical library at Museum Street. Through Barbara a large number of books and some bookcases were donated by that library to the college. Through her connections she was also able to acquire more anthroposophical books from other sources. As well as having a wide knowledge of anthroposophical books Barbara was also an expert on animal husbandry and was a recognized livestock judge. She helped Katherine Castelliz establish its beef-herd on Tablehurst Farm.

Violet Bursey came as a student during the early years at Pixton. She then took over the running of the library. Working with Barbara they created a very substantial library of around 5,000 books. Neither of them ever asked for any form of payment, in fact they both made financial donations to the college. Violet continued caring for the library for many years. She loved to see students using it and had remarkable patience with those who did not always follow procedures properly. Violet had suffered ill health for most of her childhood. I do not remember details of the problem, but as a result she had had little schooling. At some point she was taken to Rudolf Steiner and stayed for a time in Dornach. She told me once how Rudolf Steiner brought back a small dog from one of his travels and gave it to her to look after.

There were others also who assisted in the library. One of these was Justin Haynes, a former student. I remember him well as he often made donations 'for the office'. He said people giving to such organizations seldom thought about the needs of the people in the office, so he liked specially to help them. Amongst other donations was a more comfortable chair 'for the Bursar'.

Bookshop

I have already spoken of Marcia Elin when I described her and her husband Lionel in chapter 3. The bookshop could claim to be older than the college itself. Marcia was running a small 'shop' of books and Weleda products in the Sunfield Children's Homes when Emerson was founded there. When she and Lionel moved with the college to Forest Row she brought the bookshop with her. At Pixton she had it on the landing in the main house. That was, in many ways, a good place for it—though I suspect that some people were tempted to buy more books than they would read. I know I did as it was just outside my office. Later, after Ruskin was built, the bookshop was moved into a more suitable space there. In 1978, when Marcia finally retired, a former student, Eva Kulka, took it on. She had bought a house in the village in order to stay connected and to help out where she could. She ran the bookshop for some years, but I have no record of when she actually left.

When Eva finally decided to join her daughter in Australia, Kurt Falk, who had recently married Anne Stockton, offered to run it, which he did for a number of years. Then in 1985 Marie Claire Thomson, whose husband John carried responsibility for the Education Course, took over the bookshop. She ran it for the next 15 years. The turnover of the bookshop had steadily increased and was of considerable service to the students as well as generating an income for the college. All these people who ran it did so on a voluntary basis.

12
Life at the College—I

Former students have often referred to the importance of their having been at Emerson rather than to their time in a particular course. Obviously what they gained from their course studies was of prime importance, but there is no doubt about the importance also of their experience of the life of the college as a whole beyond the individual courses. Students chose, or were led, to attend a particular course and as such they learned and experienced what was to be gained in that course. Each course was an organ of the college, but it was the college as a whole that was the totality, the Being in itself. What they experienced in the life of the whole gave confirmation to what they learnt in the classroom; it entered deeply into their life of feeling and gave direction to their will forces.

The fees students paid were to attend the college not a particular course. There were only two basic tuition fees: a first year fee and second or subsequent year fee. In a similar way all staff who became members of the Association (chapter 7), as most staff did, were responsible for the whole as well as for their particular area or work. So in this chapter I shall try to say something of the life of the whole, rather than the life within any particular courses.

⋆ ⋆ ⋆

The nature of the life of the college changed and evolved over the years. Such an institution, organization or community of work has a certain organic life and evolves through the stages as any living organism does. Many of us experienced this at Emerson. But to give a description of the ongoing life as it evolved from year to year is not possible here. So, with some exceptions, I shall try to give in the main a sort of general idea as it probably was around the middle and late part of the 1970s.

But first something that Frits Julius, a teacher at The Free School in The Hague wrote:

> *When, during the Easter Teachers' Conference of 1967 at Michael Hall, Mr. Edmunds invited me to make a contribution to the work of Emerson College, I little dreamed what an adventure this would prove to be for me. In*

the Autumn term of 1968 I gave a course in Botany which meant spending five weeks in the community of the college. It was like a new world opening up for me.

In that conversation Mr. Edmunds had expressed the hope of acquiring a property for the college in the vicinity of Michael Hall. On my arrival this winter this was already an accomplished fact—an astonishingly quick development. Here at Pixton I found over 70 participants in the course, making a most harmonious community held together by strong powers of mutual sympathy. It was easy to find one's bearings. One was met on all sides with great warmth of heart.

On asking a member of the course how he felt about it all, the reply was, 'This is my real home.' This held true for many. Whoever is familiar with the situation, so riddled with doubts, in which modern young people find themselves, will also appreciate what it must mean for them to be able to speak of an environment in which they feel really at home. It was further clear what a strong sense of personal responsibility lived in them for the welfare of the whole. Conversation showed how identified they felt themselves to be with the undertaking itself. If it was criticized in any way, the immediate impulse was to defend it. This fact hangs closely together with the way the management is set up. The organization is of a kind to make the strongest appeal for individual as well as collective responsibility. Apart from the cook, the gardener, the office workers, who are inwardly related to the work, there are no employees. The general work, cleaning, preparing of vegetables, setting the tables and serving the food, care for the park surrounds, is carried by the students by their own arrangements. The greater measure of responsibility rests with the Second-Year students, but all have their share. Then there is a weekly house meeting to coordinate the various needs. Mr. Edmunds leaves these matters to the members of the course, and it can be said the household runs well and in good order.

I had the good fortune to be present at some of the study courses being given, Anthroposophy by Mr. Edmunds, Study of Man by Dr. Nunhofer, Biodynamic studies by Miss Castelliz. I can only say how greatly impressed I was by the wealth and depth of the content offered. At times one had the impression that this content was streaming down from the spiritual world there and then.

When one is accustomed to receive Anthroposophy through the Dutch and particularly through the German language, it is very interesting to hear how this declares itself through the English language. It is obvious that the German language, above all in the way Rudolf Steiner makes use of it to find the right forms of expression for what he has to convey, offers by far the best possibility of drawing near to the spiritual meaning. It is obvious that the effectiveness of the mantrams and the meditations is quite different when received in its original formulation. And yet, when one has heard a number of times an inspired presentation of the spiritual in the English language, one cannot but be deeply impressed with the exceptional quality of translucency which English has to offer. There dawns in the presence of such a community a realization of the greatness of the task of the English-speaking peoples for the spreading of Anthroposophy. One can reach, through the English language, to a sense of the great dimension of the world itself, more so than through the German language. With every translation of the books of Rudolf Steiner, one directly confronts as an Englishman or American a worldwide responsibility, for these translations extend to the greater part of the world. The vast degree of responsibility taken in a place like Emerson College becomes very clear when one meets there a man from India (Lekh Raj Ulfat), fully engaged in the course, who is himself carrying out an exceptionally rich and manifold educational and social programme in his own country, and who has become convinced that one can carry further only through the help of Rudolf Steiner's ideas. Whilst at the college there was the opportunity for a conversation with Major Ramachandra, a man of wide influence in the cultural life of India, anxious to introduce our education both with normal and retarded children as far as possible in his own country. Significant preparatory steps towards this have already been taken. The probability is that again and again people will be coming from India to train at Emerson College.

The Start of Each Year

Although most students coming to Emerson for the first time seemed to have different ideas of what they were coming to, many, if not most, found it very different from their expectations. Emerson did not easily fit into the usual idea of a college with its established procedures and ordered life, its rules and regulations, or of the kind of community of which there were many setting up in the 1960s and 70s. There was considerable freedom and lack of rules and regulations, of ordered structure into which one found one's way and needed to fit. On the other hand there was a seriousness, an assumption of each person's commitment to their search for higher truths and a morality and self-discipline by which to conduct one's life.

The beginning of each new academic year was always an exciting time. The summer work camp had ended two or three weeks before in order to

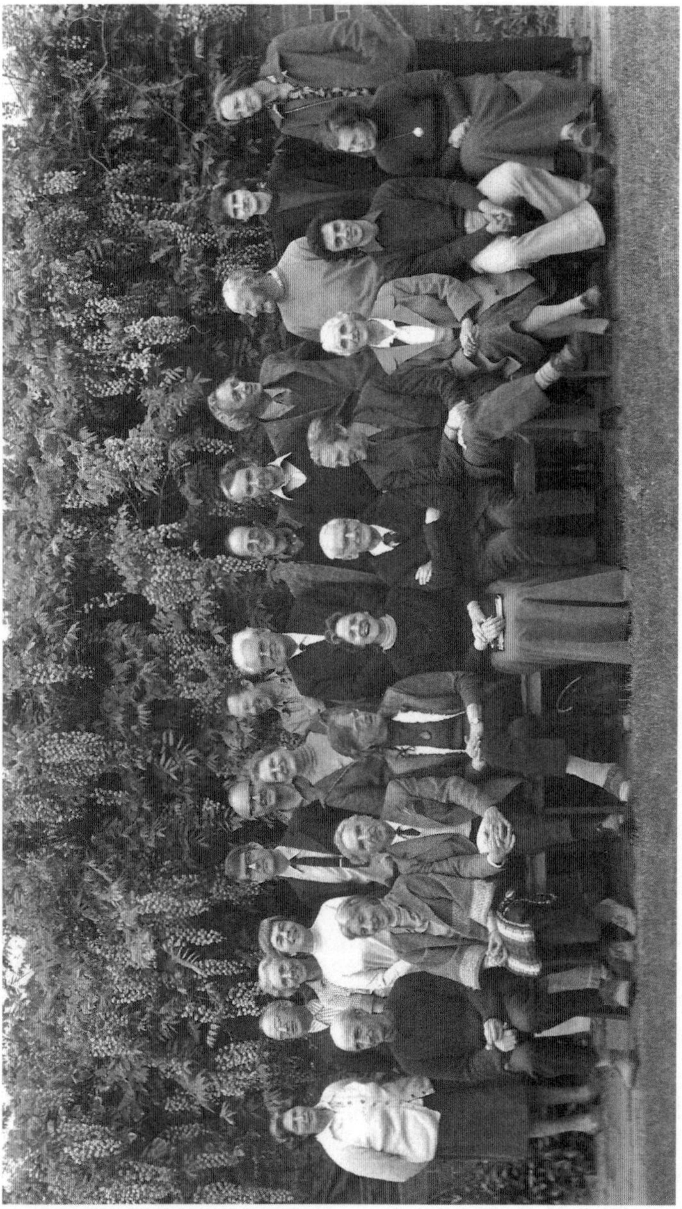

Staff, mid-1970s, back row, left to right: Myra Macdonald, Herbert Koepf, Molly von Heider, Ursula Koepf, John Davy, Michael Spence, Anne Stockton, Anthony Kaye, Fritz Koln, Peter Horsfall, Julian Pook, Ron Jarman, Alistair Macdonald, Christopher Kidman, Djobs van Houten; front row, right to left: Ilse Brice, Paul Matthews, Olive Whicher, Coen van Houten, William Mann, Roswitha Spence, Dana Prager, Francis Edmunds, Elizabeth Edmunds, John Wilkes.

create a brief, quiet, and inward time for preparation. Usually around two-thirds of the students arriving would be new, mostly for the Foundation Year. But there were always a few who went straight into the second-year training courses. Every beginning of year was different. But it was always hectic, particularly for Roswitha in the beginning, and later for Myra, Alistair, and Rachel, who were responsible for housing the students, mostly with landladies in the village. There were nearly always last-minute applications and acceptances, so more rooms would suddenly have to be found.

A number of second-year students would return early in order to help with the new arrivals. On the day the new students were due to arrive Roswitha, with a second-year helper to drive the college van, would meet each train at East Grinstead railway station. Trains then arrived hourly. So for most of the new arrivals their first meeting with Emerson was Roswitha and her driver calling out 'Anyone for Emerson College?' In her work of sorting out which student to place with which landlady, she had got to know and could remember the names and details of every student before they arrived. So she knew them immediately on their introducing themselves. This was enormously important and helpful in enabling them to feel welcomed and at home, particularly for those for whom this was a foreign country and culture.

They were then taken to Pixton where they were met by other second-year students who gave them refreshments, showed them round, and gave a first brief introduction to Emerson. Before meeting the next train Roswitha and her driver collected the previous group of new arrivals, those who would be lodged in the village, and took them to meet their landladies and settle them into their new lodging. She would also give them a map to help them find their way back to where they would have their meals. By the end of the day she could recognize and name every student who had arrived.

In the early days there was no formal registration. At the end of the day Roswitha would know who had arrived and who was still expected. Most staff and many returning students would be about the college to introduce themselves and welcome the new students. There would be an envelope for each enclosing such papers as brief information on various practical matters to help them find their way about and settle in, a timetable of the first few days, a list of all staff with their areas of responsibility, and an invoice for the fees due. A students' list would follow later—due to last minute applications and some intending students not being able to make final arrangements due to visas or financial holdups, we never knew exactly who would arrive until after the term had started. It was also surprising how often there were last-minute applications. Destiny did not always bring people along orderly paths and on time.

Over the next few days there would be a number of meetings to introduce new arrivals to the work arrangements, college functioning, members of staff, and to enable them to begin to get to know each other. They would also meet their teachers. There would be a social evening usually organized by returning students, often containing skits on aspects of the life of the college that could be extremely humorous. The students, mostly in their 20s but others ranging up even into their 60s, and from around 25 different countries and backgrounds, began to find out what they had come to. They settled in remarkably quickly. Finding themselves washing up after meals, or involved in some other domestic work, greatly helped them quickly feel at home.

The first working day, usually the Monday, always started with a whole college meeting. The opening of the new year was always special and one sensed an air of excitement and expectancy, of the beginning of a venture into unknown land. The meeting always started with a welcome. There would be some description of the coming term, of any special events, etc. An important part was the welcome from each of the Course leaders to their students with a brief description of the journey they were about to embark on. There would be some music and usually also singing. To round off the meeting, which was often light-hearted and humorous but always with a more serious undertone, it would end with a few words from Francis, John or one of the other older Course-carriers with a more reflective thought or question to carry into the term.

Over the years this opening meeting was always a powerful experience. In later years there were usually 250 or more people crowded into the room. So many new expectant faces having come along so many different paths to be here, but also former students already carrying the work out into the world who came to see the new year start and give it their good wishes. Then there were also the staff and visiting teachers and other friends of the college or of the students. To see all these people, all in one way or another brought together and touched, often very profoundly, by this work that originated out of the wisdom and impulse of one man—Francis Edmunds—this could move one very deeply.

The Events of the Year

At the beginning and end of each term the whole community always met to open and close the term together. The opening meeting would include a welcome to any new courses, students or staff. There would be some sort of looking back to any interesting events or developments at Pixton during the holiday, and to any interesting travels or events anyone had experienced. There would then be a look at the coming term, some music and singing and a thought to take into the term.

The closing meeting would be somewhat similar but much of it in reverse.

The Michaelmas Festival on 29 September was the first event after the start of the new year. For most, a Michaelmas Festival was something quite new to their experience, so time had to be found before the event to introduce the significance and importance of the festivals.

The Christian Festivals of Michaelmas, Christmas, Easter, and Whitsun that we would celebrate during the year played an essential part in the experience of the cycle of the year at Emerson. Elizabeth Edmunds took primary responsibility for organizing them. In later years individual Courses themselves took responsibility for one or other festival, but during the early years they were very much college affairs. For each festival Elizabeth would invite a few carefully chosen students, not from any particular Course, to prepare the festival with her. She would not necessarily choose those with experience of the festival, or even a connection to Christianity. She had a remarkable intuitive ability to find those students who had an inner question, perhaps still unconscious, to that particular festival, or were on a search for what could be found in it. She would leave much of the arranging of the festival to this group, she herself helping with the study and possibly making suggestions or comments on their ideas.

The festivals varied but were nearly always very special occasions. They usually included eurythmy and/or music and on most occasions a talk by one of the students as well as one by a teacher. It was remarkable how often, in their simple and often hesitant way, what the student brought was listened to with greater attention; not because what they had to say came out of any greater wisdom, but because they had clearly struggled to achieve what they did—they had come a greater distance. My memory is of many deeply moving festivals through which much understanding of what was being celebrated shone through. Except where the festival fell in the holidays they were always celebrated on the actual date of the festival, whichever day of the week that was.

Festivals were always treated differently from other events. There was usually some sort of introduction to each at a House Meeting just before the actual event. We tried to maintain the awareness that they were not entertainment, nor educational in the usual sense. They were something one participated in. Even if one only listened to a talk or watched a play, one tried to live into and experience what stood behind the event, its meaning and place in the whole course of human evolution. The hall was specially decorated and we came into the room and sat down quietly without the usual chatter, no photography, and no applause after any contribution.

For many students, even many brought up in a Christian tradition, these festivals led to an experience of something of the Christ event very different and on a far deeper level than is usually portrayed in the Christian churches. It sowed the seeds of questions in many students that awakened a need to know and understand more. For others it was experienced as a challenge to their accustomed accepted beliefs. Though these festivals played an important and ongoing part in the life of the college, there were often others. Students from different cultures and religions would sometimes arrange festivals from their own traditions. These could be beautiful occasions and were always welcomed and supported.

The International Evening was usually placed during the first half of the autumn term. This was one of the highlights of the year and revealed the richness of the international spread of the college. It was held early in the year while students still had something about them of the culture out of which they had come—before they had dropped this and become more distinctly individual human beings. The idea was that students from each country would get together and present something of their country or culture. It could be anything they liked, serious or funny, poem, song or skit. The evening was always very special and popular. Items were often extremely funny, sometimes very serious or emotional, occasionally awful.

The Three Advent Festivals (the fourth normally came after term ended) were very special in the dawning sense of the coming of the light—the

Christ light in the child born on the night of Christmas Eve. This was symbolized in the lighting of the candles increasing from one on the first to four on the fourth Sunday of Advent. In preparation for the festival there would have been a making of Advent wreaths, usually as an evening activity. Annemarie always took a large part in organizing this. On each of the Advent Sundays there would be a festival, usually short and in the morning.

On later occasions the Education Course organized the festival as it was often done in the schools. On entering the room everyone received an unlighted candle sometimes placed into an apple. After we had all assembled in a circle with our unlighted candles we were led into an inward spiral to a point in the middle where there was a lighted candle, often placed at the foot of an Angel Being, from which we each lit our candle. Then with our lighted candles we continued back in an outward spiral between the forms of the inward spiral. It was a very special and deeply moving experience to be involved in such an event.

With health and safety regulations as they are today such an event would probably not be possible. As someone then carrying some responsibility for safety, I remember thinking at the time, with the naked and unprotected flames and some people's loose clothing and long hair, was this too dangerous and should we stop it? But I remember also the sense of a spiritual presence, that as long as there was no fear, only trust in the Spirit, then only what lay in people's destiny could come about.

The Christmas Plays also came at this time. Instead of the Oberufer plays normally performed for the children by the teachers in Waldorf schools, Francis Edmunds had adapted the English Coventry cycle of plays to the needs of the adult students of the college. As an extracurricular activity outside the Courses Francis would work with those students who chose to take part with him to put on the Paradise, Shepherds, and Kings plays. Occasionally, instead of the Paradise play they would perform, mainly in eurythmy, the story of Seth, the third son of Adam and Eve. Working with him included coming to some understanding of the meaning of the plays. Something of this was also explained to the college before the plays were performed. These plays brought many students and staff into actual active involvement in the Christmas mood.

The Christmas Festival was really a sort of preparatory festival because Christmas, of course, would be after term ended. It was usually on the last evening of term and had two parts: the Christmas Festival and the Christmas Social Evening and included a candle-lit Christmas tree.

The Social Evening followed the Christmas Festival, sometimes with community supper for everyone in between. These social evenings varied from year to year but there were generally three events in them which I think can indicate something of their character. One was the giving of presents; those who wanted to, which was usually almost every one, before the event put their names in a box; then we all took a name out; we made, found or bought a special present for that person. This meant thinking about that person, quietly observing and getting to know something about them. The presents were put under the Christmas tree and at some point in the evening given out to the person named on them. The presents were usually given anonymously.

Another special event started one year when we had a number of young women from Scandinavia. They performed the coming of the light in the entry of Santa Lucia and her procession. This is traditionally celebrated in the Scandinavian countries on the 13 December. First we all stood in a great circle round the edges of the room, each holding an unlighted candle. Most of the electric lights were turned off so the room was darkened. Then from outside we heard the voices of women singing. The door was opened and Santa Lucia dressed in white with a crown of lighted candles on her head and followed by a procession of women also dressed in white and each holding a lighted candle, slowly entered the room singing the traditional Santa Lucia song. As they passed round the room we each lit our candle from them. Slowly the room lightened until sometimes well over 150 candles shone out into the room. It was always a very beautiful and moving event.

The third very popular event was when Francis Edmunds read from Charles Dickens's Christmas Carol. He usually read the part where the ghost first appears to Scrooge. It was always a brilliant and very funny performance and had everyone in fits of laughter.

Christmas and the 13 Holy Nights, from Christmas Eve to Epiphany, were celebrated during the Christmas holiday. Many students, particularly those who could not go home, would stay on to experience this, or at least part of it. Each night there would be a lighting of the Tree—only candles were used, never electric lights. Then there might be a short talk from someone, a reading on a Christmas theme or some artistic activity.

Sometimes there were other activities such as candle-making. There would usually be singing or music and then refreshments. Finally there would be an extinguishing of the candles. The whole celebration was always a quiet and inward event. On Epiphany, 6 January, there would be a small celebration for those still at the college. This would take place in the morning.

The Spring Term—some preferred to call it the winter term. This was for many a more testing period. Not only was it outwardly a dark, cold, and damp time—particularly for those from warmer climates—but especially for Foundation Year students, it could be a difficult time inwardly when they experienced acute loneliness and being thrown back on themselves. As one student put it: in the first term the old forms of support that gave a sense of security were shown to be not what they seemed. In the second term many felt directionless and unsure of themselves. It was often not till the third that they found their new directions and sense of purpose.

The Carnival was always welcomed as a relief coming during this more difficult period. After that first one in 1968 mentioned in chapter 6 it became an annual event. There was a different theme each year and most people came in fancy dress. The carnival was a time to relax, to put aside the serious aspects of life and enjoy oneself, to let oneself go. They nearly always included skits, often including one by the staff.

The Easter Festival, really a preparation for Easter, came at the end of the spring term, Easter itself falling during the holidays.

The Emerson Italy Art Tour, started by William Mann in 1965 and described in chapter 3, was usually organized for the Easter holidays. With William's support Julian Pook took these on. For those students who took part these were rich and soul-nourishing experiences.

The Summer Term

The Mayfair early in the summer term was a time when the college opened itself to the wider village community. As described in chapter 6 the first Mayfair was in 1968. Since then it has been held every year and has become popular with many children of the wider community. The weather has not always been kind to us, but only once did the fair have to be brought inside. The Maypole dancing, the central attraction for many, always attracted a large audience. It was wonderful to see when at the end all the children were invited to join in. The fact that there was no amplification or recorded music—everything was live and human scale—made the event different and special for many.

The Whitsun Festival This festival, celebrated on the seventh Sunday after Easter, usually fell around the middle of the summer term. Francis often said that he felt that Emerson College had a particular connection to the Whitsun Festival. The coming of the Holy Spirit in the form of the mighty rushing wind and of the tongues of fire that descended on each of Christ's Apostles as they sat in the upper room at Pentecost was a forerunner of, or a preparation for, the awakening of the free human spirit within the individual human being. This awakening was central to the task of the Foundation Year.

One regular feature of the festival was to have the relevant part of the bible read out in many different languages by students from those countries. This was always a moving experience.

The Shakespeare Plays directed by Francis Edmunds, were one of the main features of the summer term. They were college events and many students and staff, sometimes up to 60 or 70 were, in one way or other, involved in them, either on- or back-stage. While Francis directed them the plays always included eurythmy and music. Elizabeth worked with students to develop special eurythmy performances appropriate to the plays. While the main activity was extracurricular and participation open to any student interested, much of the making of the costumes and scenery was done as a craft activity within the Foundation Year. Roswitha, after her earlier training, had worked with the Royal Shakespeare Theatre in Stratford-upon-Avon and with English National Opera. So, working closely with and learning from Francis, with teams of students she was able to bring her professional expertise to the designing and making of the costumes and scenery. In these classes she showed how, through the careful use of colour, texture and style, the costumes could bring to light something of the character's soul journey within the play. She would go to jumble sales and such events buying old curtains, bedspreads, and similar used material. These made good costumes as they did not look too new, and they were cheap. Over the years the college acquired in this way a very considerable wardrobe for future plays.

For many involved in the acting, working with Francis was a powerful and awakening experience. But in whatever way they were involved, whether with the costumes, scenery, lighting, music, eurythmy or publicity, students were brought into involvement with the deeper meaning of the plays, and to experience something of their wisdom. In fact, so many were involved that something of this tended to permeate the whole college.

Francis himself put an enormous amount of time and energy into these plays. Rehearsals were normally in the evenings. Even after a day of teaching and dealing with correspondence, interviews etc. he would keep them working, sometimes till beyond midnight. There were usually two performances for the college, one for the immediate community and the second for family and friends. The third was a public performance. Despite the difficulty of understanding Shakespeare spoken by many of our foreign students these plays were very popular and gained a reputation for excellence. But there was almost always a period of crisis just before first night when many, particularly Francis and Roswitha, said it was not good enough for a public performance. But the fact that those involved had worked hard to understand the deep human truths shone through and always lifted the play. Everyone was full of congratulations. They were performed during the last week or 10 days of the term.

Francis carried main responsibility for these plays until he finally retired at the end of the year 1976–7. At that time they were also taken into the curriculum of the Foundation Year. Ursula Koepf produced them for the next two years and then Dawn Langman took over the drama work in the Course.

The St John's Fire was the final event of the year before the students left, many to return the following year, but most, particularly of the training courses, to step back into the wider world and take up their work or to continue training elsewhere. It was for many a special time, a time to look back on new discoveries, on a change of course or of transformation and a new beginning, and on new friends. It was also a time to say goodbye to so many friends with whom important connections had been forged through shared experiences. But a deeper understanding of what they had been through would usually come later.

The end of the year could be very cramped but exhilarating with the

Shakespeare plays, final course exhibitions, presentations and farewell parties, a final college social evening, and the St John's Festival and Fire.

* * *

Music This played an important part in the life of the college from the beginning. In 1971 Julian Pook joined the staff as a music teacher. Much of his work was extracurricular. When there were enough students he ran a small orchestra. He also conducted a choir for those who wanted to sing, which usually was many. He arranged musical contributions for many of the events of the year such as the plays, maypole dancing, etc. Individual contributions were encouraged for instance for the start and ending of the House Meetings. He also arranged concerts by invited artists. These were open to the public and became an important feature in the life of the wider community. Once a year there was a concert given solely by Emerson College musicians.

There were also occasional special music workshops such as the one reported by John Davy in the Progress Report of 1977:

> *A special highlight of the year was the Bach week which opened our Spring Term after Easter, initiated by Miha Pogacnik, and organised with the help of Julian Pook and a number of local musicians. There were seven concerts, progressing from two evenings of unaccompanied violin works, through a sonata evening, then two evenings devoted to the Art of Fugue. Finally, there was a cantata evening, and an orchestral evening including a violin concerto and a Brandenberg concerto.*
>
> *It was a very rich and moving experience, and there was a special power in the evenings for the art of fugue. This work, Bach's last, was introduced by another visitor, Herr Schriefer, (whose main work is to carry forward a new impulse in singing which comes from Rudolf Steiner through Frau Werbeck, but who is also a profound scholar and historian of music.) He showed how Bach had woven into this work a relationship to the world evolutionary process. There was a deep stillness in the hall as the last—unfinished—fugue ended in the middle of a bar, the moment which marks Bach's death.*
>
> *Among a group of people striving to live their way through a whole year into a deeper apprehension of the nature and destiny of humanity, such moments born out of the arts have a special strength. We are deeply grateful to Miha Pogacnik for what he brought, for his beautiful playing, and to Herr Schriefer for the great enrichment he offered.*

Julian left the college in 1983 and much of his work of carrying the musical impulse was taken over by Ursula Koepf, who brought her own particular genius to the task. Under her guidance the number of concerts grew.

Extracurricular Studies

Through the year there were at different times evening lectures and study groups offered. These were not Course-orientated but, like the choir, were for anyone wishing to attend. Probably the best known of these was William Mann on History of Art. These were weekly lectures which he gave for many years, and were an inspiration for many students and were always well attended, including by people from the wider locality. They, of course, reflected and illuminated from a different perspective what John Davy gave the Foundation Year in his lectures on the evolution of consciousness. Like John, William had the ability to bring the subject alive for his students in a remarkable and inspiring way.

Visitors

Through the year, but particularly during the summer there was a constant stream of visitors. The growing Emerson soon developed a reputation as an interesting place to visit and many leading anthroposophical friends when travelling to England from different parts of the world would make a point of visiting. I remember a young woman from the auditor's office sitting in my office checking the books (that was before we had computers). Looking up after a visitor had just left me she said 'Sitting here is like sitting in the middle of the world, with people coming from all over.' Such visitors were often asked to say something of their work at the House Meeting, or to give a lecture.

There were others, often leaders in their particular fields of anthroposophical work, and also individual members of the Vorstand of the Anthroposophical Society in Dornach, who were invited to give lecture courses or workshops at the college. On some occasions this was given to the whole college or even opened to the local community. Such visitors always seemed to enjoy coming and working with the students. They seemed to like especially the freer culture of the college, and the lack of any VIP status.

Then there were other periodic visitors such as Richard St Barbe

Baker, author of *Man of the Trees*.* He planted the tulip tree in the lawn outside the kitchen. Two others were Ernst Friedrich (E.F.) Schumacher, the economist who developed the ideas of appropriate technologies and author of *Small is Beautiful*,† and Laurens van der Post the humanitarian, conservationist, and writer, particularly on African peoples.

* Richard St Barbe Baker and Karen Gridley, *Man of the Trees* (Willits CA: Ecology Action, 1989).

† E.T. Schumacher, *Small is Beautiful* (London: Vintage, 1993).

13
Life at the College—II

Joann Ianniello wrote of her experience in the Social Development Centre, including one term in the Teacher-training Course at Pixton, during the year 1978–9:

> *The time spent at Emerson College and the Centre for Social Development has deep meaning for me. The cooperative learning experience and the way we were taught as adults was very special. I suppose it is the meeting each other on a soul level that has stayed with me all these years.*
>
> *I am fortunate to still be in communication with friends that I made while at Emerson.*
>
> *Today, as I celebrated Michaelmas, I reflected on how the festivals and the seasons of the year came to have more meaning to my life after being a student at Emerson. I still can recall singing 'Sleepers Awake' for the Michaelmas gathering. The group who attended the Centre sang under the direction of Anne Tyler. 'Forging the Future' is perhaps the main reason for the existence of Emerson College. It is a portal for the work of Anthroposophy to enter into the earth's stream. Students from all over the world are drawn to come to Emerson and meet on a soul level which continues to carry one forward in one's incarnation. The impulse for Emerson College, begun by Francis and Elizabeth Edmunds, still has a purpose and meaning for today's world. 'Encountering of Soul' meeting your own Soul and those of others is the deeper meaning behind all the lectures at Emerson. One of the songs we sang at the Centre: 'And we dug right down to the bottom of our Souls to see what we had inside.' still resonates in me 33 years later!*
>
> *After leaving Emerson, it was very strange to adjust back to life in NYC! I can remember standing in my local supermarket and feeling that 'none of the foods are real in this supermarket'. After a year of biodynamic foods under the skill of Wendy Cook, the foods at my local supermarket were a shadow of what I had experienced at Emerson. The whole milk in the milk carton could not compare to the delicious milk from the cows at Old Plaw Hatch Farm!!!! It was like liquid vanilla ice cream!*

An International College

Emerson College was always intended to be an international college in England, not a British college for the British with some from other countries. As already indicated Francis had a particular connection to America and at one time thought of founding the college there. But he told me once that it was particularly important that Americans met the European culture in Europe, and an international college would have to be in the English language. In America it would never really be international, especially at that time with the exchange rate as it was. So it had to be in England.

Its international nature was part of what made it so special for many students. At the beginning around 25 per cent of the students were British, but by the mid-1980s this figure had fallen to between 15 per cent and 20 per cent. Each year from 1970 until 1986 there were more from America than from Britain, and from 1984 to 1986 there were actually more Germans than British. Up until 1986 students had come from 46 different countries. These figures are based on student numbers including the Priest Training and the Social Development Centre. The proportion of British in the Foundation Year and on Pixton campus was lower, usually around 15 per cent. So Emerson could truly claim to be an international college, not a British one with some foreign students. Though not to the same extent, quite a number of the staff also came from other countries.

Due to this international mix, students came to experience, many quite strongly and for the first time, the one humanity nature of world humanity and over against this the unique and individual nature of each human being. In our time, as evolved out of the past, each human being is primarily a separate and unique individual. Only secondly can they rightly be looked at as of a particular race, religion or sex. To see and take an interest in only those who are like oneself leads to nationalism, to what was right for humanity in the past. To be interested in and come to love those who are different from oneself leads to a recognition of and a love for all humanity. That is the way into the future.

Community

The college never set out to be a community as such. In the early 1970s the word 'community' was widely used by many of the younger generation. Francis was always wary of this term. He once explained to a group of us that there were two things in life which one did not have to concern oneself with; they came of their own accord. One was death. The other was community—if a group of people came together to carry out a work for a purpose beyond themselves community arose of itself.

True community would never come about when worked for as an aim in itself.

The social life, the festivals and the carrying of the daily domestic work were all part of the learning social experience of Emerson College. The carrying of the domestic work may have saved money and helped keep the fees low, but that was not its primary purpose. As I mentioned in chapter 8, the working together, doing work for the benefit of the community, was an important balance to the course work. The rhythmic alternation between these two activities formed a breathing in and breathing out within the social life of the college.

But the community work did not originally come about with this in mind, or only partially so. A clearer consciousness of this came later. It originally came about more as an organic development out of the early years of the college. For the first five years, of necessity, Francis left much of the organizing of the domestic arrangements and the cleaning and upkeep of the buildings to the students themselves. Even as the college grew and moved to the run-down wooden huts in Forest Row, there was no maintenance or housekeeping staff. As described earlier, it was part of the life of this early pioneering period that students organized and themselves did the cleaning and much of the maintenance. Until later when more staff joined there was no one else to do this—Francis himself already carried an immense workload; and also, in this sense, he was not a practical man.

For many years after the move to Pixton the students themselves continued to carry responsibility for planning and organizing the domestic work. This was usually done by second-year students who passed responsibility for it on to first-year students early in the new year. The actual organization varied over the years, but generally everyone had two jobs, one around the meals and one of more general housekeeping or environmental work. For meals, tables had to be set up before the meal and after the meal plates and cutlery cleared and washed, tables cleaned and floors swept. All plates and cutlery had to be put through the washing machine, dried and put away. Pots and pans were washed by hand. All students and some staff were put into teams mixed across the courses, one team for each day of the week. Early morning vegetable preparation and the many weakly cleaning jobs were generally allocated by Course. I remember one older student we had. She was a retired headmistress of a State school. Now here she was at Emerson, doing her share of cleaning the tables and sweeping the floor. On one occasion she paused in her work and said: 'If my teachers could see me now they would not believe this.'

In the early years there was also one afternoon per week allocated for garden work. That afternoon there were no classes and everyone was meant to contribute to the upkeep of the environment. But while many valued this time working physically in the environment doing community work, there were always others who used the time to go shopping or fulfilling other personal needs. Through the year numbers always declined and after trying a number of different forms the arrangement was eventually discontinued.

Each year there were two or three workdays, for example on the farm harvesting the potatoes or carrots, or on the college campus in the late autumn sweeping up all the fallen leaves to clear the roads and footpaths and to provide compost for the gardens. On these days all classes were cancelled and everyone, students and staff, joined in the work. These were important times when people found they could meet each other on a quite different level than in normal college life. A student might find her or himself picking potatoes alongside, for example, a teacher from another Course. Community was experienced in a real sense in working together at a common task. On the farm workdays the kitchen would usually provide a communal picnic meal out on the fields.

Regular classes normally finished around four or five o'clock. But in the evenings there were frequently extracurricular activities such as choir, lectures from interesting people visiting the college, and study groups on different subjects not necessarily connected to any particular Course. These were often arranged by the college, but were on occasion asked for, or arranged by the students themselves. All this on top of the normal course-work sometimes led to students doing too much and then having to drop out of some activities. The danger was of what we called spiritual indigestion.

I always found an intense but tranquil beauty in walking through the campus in the evening and, hearing, coming from one or other room, the sound of a piano being played, or the choir singing, or some other activity such as the clack of the looms in the weavery. Robert Koerber, a student in 1972 who later became involved in founding and running the bakery (chapter 17), remembered:

> *After dinner and clean up, people would drift into the kitchen around 10pm, waiting for Francis (Edmunds) to drift in around 10:30pm, looking for warm*

milk before going to bed. He was enthroned on the bouncy stool near the stove and then the students would gather around. Prosper and Christa Nebel, Harm Huizinga, Beverly Kennedy, Lori Patterson, Tom Hammond, Keith Morris, John Platt and others drifting in and out would start open-ended discussions with Francis. Sometimes Francis would grab the shoulder of someone and ask 'What's bothering you?'. When we asked 'What will our work be in the world when we leave the college?' he often said, 'Create your own work. Start a school, create something'.

When Edmunds spoke with you, you were the only person in the room. People stood as equals when talking with him, in a way that you remembered.

When this smaller group let him talk, he often could say things that he couldn't say in a larger group. Out of the Parsifal Course, the important thing was not getting the chalice but instead the process of getting there.

House Meeting

Every week there was a House Meeting (many years later it was renamed the College Meeting). This was a particularly important meeting in the life of the college. It was the one time in the week when the whole college, including families and visitors, could meet. It fulfilled many functions. It was a time when information could be shared such as proposals for future activities and reports on past events or from courses on their work. Visitors would be introduced. Someone who had been travelling or had been to an interesting event outside the college might report on it. Also problems within the social or domestic life of the college could be brought and discussed and a solution looked for—the problem of coffee cups being left around was one that lasted through all the years. Anyone could bring a concern, report or a proposal for a new initiative to the meeting. Matters were often brought in the form of skits, which were sometimes extremely hilarious. It was a time when the college also kept in touch with and discussed current world events. Students from parts of the world where such events were unfolding could share interesting insights.

The House Meeting was also a time where college events such as festivals or the Mayfair could be prepared. It often included music or the whole college singing. Francis sometimes spoke of the importance of all the college singing together. The meeting played an essential role in both the social and educational life and so it was generally scheduled within the normal working week. Originally Francis Edmunds himself ran these meetings, but later they were taken over by students, sometimes with a staff member.

But the House Meeting had another particularly important function. There was that which, of necessity, divided people from each other: the division between students, teachers and administrative staff, between the different courses, and between the different departments and functions. Some people through their capacities and wisdom were particularly important within the whole while others fulfilled only minor roles. It was in the House Meeting that these divisions were overcome and all people seen as equal members of the Emerson community. All people would be listened to with equal interest. It was always moving how someone new and inexperienced, hesitatingly telling us for example about an event in his or her home country, would be listened to with the same attention as would be given to an older more experienced teacher; or someone just learning a new musical instrument and persuaded to play to us would be listened to and willed on through their mistakes with real attention and love. These were often greatly moving and powerful unifying experiences within the community.

It was really in the House Meeting that each became aware of and connected to the whole, rather than their own small part of the college. In many ways an important aspect, particularly of the Foundation Year, was this becoming aware of and connecting to the larger community beyond oneself, to humanity as a whole rather than each to his own little separate world. But there were no rules, no one had to attend. It could only truly function when it was willed by each individual, it had to come out of each one's self discipline—this itself was educational.

Of course, there were always some, both staff and students, who tended to drop out, particularly if there was too much business and not enough of an interesting and soul-nourishing nature. But those who did not attend could not be full members of the community; they could not know what was going on nor enter into the full life of the college.

Student Housing

For the first two years at Pixton there was virtually no accommodation for students on campus. The first student accommodation, two student houses each with eight single rooms, was completed in September 1969. Rooms for most students had to be found in the village. Forest Row then had a population of around 4,000, so landladies offering rooms were few and difficult to find. It greatly helped that the Christian Community had recently purchased a large old house—Shalesbrooke—for a Priest Training Centre. They had spare rooms and were glad to house some of our students—this helped both institutions. The majority of students came from abroad and it was not easy for them to find rooms for themselves on arrival so the college found and rented the rooms, and placed the students in them. This arrangement meant that the college was able to build up a good relationship with the landladies, giving them greater security and so securing the rooms for future students. Roswitha took responsibility for this; finding rooms, placing the students, and working with and maintaining good relations with the landladies which often included sorting out problems between them and the students.

As the college grew every year there was an continuing increase in students needing accommodation. Frequently, sometimes at the last minute, Francis would accept a late applicant and Roswitha, or later Myra, had to somehow find another room, persuading some village householder of the joys of having an Emerson student in their house. This involvement with the local community did give the college a very real connection with the local village community. Some students actually preferred to live off campus with a local family, and some landladies loved having students from different parts of the world and kept up a connection even after the students had left.

The lack of student housing created a number of other challenges. With few exceptions the rooms with landladies did not include meals or cooking facilities, so all meals were provided at Pixton. This meant that most students came up from their room in the village, which could be a mile away, before breakfast and stayed on campus until, often, late at night. During this time they did not have access to any small quiet space of their own unless they went back to their room. This was a very real problem, particularly for some. We tried to alleviate the situation, but each year the numbers increased as more and more people wanted to join the college. But they understood the problem and somehow survived with little complaint. Few felt that what they gained from the college should be denied to others just so that they themselves had more space. This situation was, of course, not created intentionally, but the gaining of patience and equanimity in facing hindrances and overcoming difficulties was part of the inner path of development that was central to the Foundation Year work, though perhaps not so much a part of second-year studies. Nothing worthwhile in life is gained without struggle, and looking back I do believe this was part of the struggle of life at Emerson that helped many gain so much. As more accommodation with cooking facilities was later built on campus something of this was lost.

Meals

Three meals a day 365 days a year were provided by Anthony Kaye and his helpers, and later by those who followed. Meals always started with a grace followed by the announcing of the menu. Only after that was the meal served. There was always vegetarian food and two or three days a week there was also a meat dish. The meal ended with a cooked sweet. Coffee or various teas were available after the meal. As the farm developed and the college vegetable gardens were established the proportion of the food that came from our own sources increased dramatically. It was always intended, or hoped, that students would have their meals at the college. There were two important reasons for this. Firstly, it insured that students regularly ate adequate and healthy food. As I indicated in chapter 3 Francis recognized the importance of healthy food for young people setting out on the sort of work they would be doing at Emerson College. At that time there was little general recognition of the importance of the quality of food in the wider world. (I look at certain financial implications of this in chapter 16).

Secondly, the sharing of meals in community, particularly lunches, was an important part of the life of the college. There was no hierarchy or other division in the dining rooms. It was a time when staff and students from the different courses and areas of work, mixed with each other on a free human basis. Many important visiting lecturers, coming from more structured institutions, loved this; as one said to me 'At Emerson there are no VIPs.' At the beginning, with few exceptions, the whole college community met at lunch time. There were no meal tickets or other checking as to who had or had not paid. It was part of the learning experience of the college that it was assumed that anyone who had opted out of paying for meals would not have one. Of course there were at least two of us in the office who might recognize if someone was having a meal who should not be, then we would raise the question with him or her, but that seldom happened. In the early days, there was a rotating team of students who served the meal. They would come to the table and ask each person what he or she would like, and then bring it to them. Later this evolved to someone from each table collecting what the others wanted, then later to each getting it for him or herself. There were also times when each table had their own dishes from which to help themselves.

There were also occasions during the year, normally four, when a festive meal would be served for the whole college, including families. Two regular occasions were Christmas and Whitsun. The Whitsun meal was usually served outside on the lawn. These meals were considered as part of the life of the college so were not charged for under board and lodging.

Space became a problem as numbers increased. There came a time when it was necessary for certain other spaces, particularly the Education Course room and the wooden hut, to double up as dining room spaces.

Crèche and Mothers' Group

During the 1970s there were many families with very young children who came to the college. In 1970–71 there were 12 families with the father attending the college, two with the mother attending, and six mothers attending while their children were at school. Coming to the college was an enormous undertaking for these people. They were mostly from America where the advantageous exchange rate of that time did make it easier, but it was still a very great expense. Some had had to rent out or even sell their home in America and rent one here in England for the two years that they usually intended to stay.

At the college we did not feel it right or spiritually healthy that one parent should gain all the soul nourishment that the college had to offer while the other in looking after the children and home was denied this. We therefore offered that in all such family situations where one partner was a full-time student, the other would be welcomed to attend all Foundation Year morning courses. These ran each weekday from 8.30 to 10 am. In order to make this possible Rachel Horsfall offered to run a crèche for the children too young to go to school. She ran this in Pixton, in the long, or north, dining rooms. She sometimes had up to 12 children to look after. So the students quickly became accustomed to sharing their space with very young children during coffee break! This possibility—enabling mothers or fathers to join in and benefit from what the college offered—was enormously important for them and would strengthen the family life in the future. There were no charges for this; it was felt that the families had already committed themselves to enough expense.

At the same time Gudrun Davy started meeting with the mothers, forming a parents' group that met weekly to discuss the many questions that arose in bringing up young children. It enabled them also to learn something of what anthroposophy had to offer concerning young children and family life.

Weddings

Destiny brought individual young people to the college for many different purposes. Some found here their future life partners. In those early days it was unthinkable for anyone to have their wedding anywhere other than amongst their friends, or 'family', at Emerson. The college was always happy to host such occasions and many student friends joined with the kitchen in preparing a meal and the festivities. Probably most actual weddings took place in the Christian Community Chapel, then in Ashurstwood, with the reception and festivities afterwards at Emerson. But some devised their own words and celebrated it in the college, or in the college gardens. Once there was a Jewish wedding. The couple found a rabbi from London who was willing to conduct the ceremony in the eurythmy house. He was a remarkable and interesting man who occasionally paused the ceremony to explain the form and reason for certain aspects of it. I found it very enlightening, especially in marriage being an affair of the community, not just of the two people being married. In most years there was at least one wedding, but often many more. Roswitha, having amongst other jobs worked at one time for a London couturier, made the bride's dress for most weddings as her gift to the couple.

Television, Alcohol, and Drugs

There was no television or radio provided by the college. If students wanted it they had to provide it for themselves. The college did not, of course, forbid a student to watch television—that had to be a free choice—but it set out to be a place where a person who chose to could, for a time, withdraw from the stresses, demands and technology of the wider world into a quieter place in order to struggle with those inner questions to which they had come to find answers. For most students, though with varying degrees of consciousness, this was a time when they chose to put aside the world from which they had just come in order to find new purpose in their lives and to awaken those intentions they had resolved upon before birth—not to run from the outer world, but to gather strength in order to later return to work within it. For similar reasons alcohol and drugs were not tolerated in the college. Again, it was not actually forbidden that a student should drink alcohol, but it was understood that they worked counter to what the college set out to provide for the student just as an athlete would understand that certain drugs and stimulants worked against what he aspired to achieve. The freedom of the student to run his life as he chose had, of course, to be respected, but the college also had a right to the freedom to choose not to work with a person who took drugs.

There were always newspapers supplied to the common room; generally two copies of each of four or five English and international quality papers.

College Growth

As I have already described, the college began in 1962 with the one course—what was later called the Foundation Year. In 1984–5, 22 years later there were 10 full-time courses plus the independent studies programme running at Pixton and the Social Development Course at Old Plaw Hatch. As far as I can ascertain the numbers for 1984–5 can be given as:

Foundation Year	74
Education	41
Agriculture	23
Sculpture	16
Education Eurythmy	17
Rural Development	11
Voice	11
Witten Annen English Language	15
Speech and Drama	11
Independent Programmes	4
Total at Pixton	223
Social Development Centre	35
Grand Total	258

It might also help to form an idea of the international nature of the college if I give some idea of the 23 countries from which the students came during the year 1984–5:

USA	59
Germany	54
UK	49
Australia and New Zealand	18
Canada	14
Holland	8
Rest of Europe (12 countries)	34
Israel	7

South America	8
Asia	3
Africa	4

With some fluctuations overall student numbers at Pixton had steadily increased over the years until in 1984–5 there was a larger than usual increase. From then on there was, again with fluctuations, a slow but steady decrease. But the increased numbers together with the increase in courses had created considerable difficulties. The shortage of study spaces of all kinds and of student housing were serious problems. In 1984 there were far fewer study spaces available than there are now. The present Flowform building, Biodynamic Agriculture building, and Red Art Studio had not yet been built.

The larger Courses often had to divide for study groups and for arts and crafts, so adding to the number of spaces needed. Additionally most Courses wanted their students to do eurythmy at least once and sometimes twice per week—they nearly all wanted this at the same time—between coffee and lunch. It was an enormous work of juggling to fit everything into the few suitable spaces. Timetables had to be programmed around the availability of such spaces. Peter Horsfall took on this task; I do not think anyone else could have done it. He had the clear thinking, organizing ability, as well as the quiet diplomacy to deal with teachers who had their own demands. There were also times when students and/or teachers needed a space for a special meeting or study. Patiently he tried always to fit these in.

14
Former Students Write

I give below extracts from letters or emails received from former students—not in any particular order—which I think will be of interest.

Anne Cook (1973–6)

Dear Michael,

Craig and I attended a two-year training in Biodynamics from September 1973 to July 1975. The first year we were apprentices on Old Plaw Hatch Farm and came to Pixton House 1/2 day/ week for classes with Dr. Koepf, John Docherty and Molly von Heider. We stayed for dinner and attended readings by Katherine Castelliz. There were 10 apprentices in this program: four from Plaw Hatch, four from Busses Farm and two from Tablehurst. Emerson provided student visas. That half day of teaching was so important during an otherwise extremely difficult year at Plaw Hatch. Manning had just bought it and was unsure what he was doing. Tuesday afternoons were a lifeline for us.

The following September, 1974, we started on the Agricultural Course with the largest group ever till that point (19). We were in the little hut next to the kitchen. Many of us fell asleep for lack of oxygen, but for much of the year we couldn't open the windows because all we had for heat was a two-bar electric fire. We had Dr. Koepf every day, John Davy, Walter Rudert, John Docherty and Annemarie Vinkhuyzen for ongoing practical courses. We had eurythmy with Elizabeth Edmunds and Roger Yates, choir with Julian Pook, speech with Graham Rickett and projects with different mentors. In the spring, Craig went to work on a horse farm in Coleman's Hatch, but I stayed and finished the training. We joined the rest of the school for House Meetings, festivals, plays and performances.

From 75–76 I was in the second group of eurythmy training, which was only one year for us. We had Roger and Christopher Kidman, and Molly when she returned from New Zealand in March. We had Julian for music, speech with a fantastic German lady (farmer's wife from Canterbury), modelling with John Wilkes, gardening with Annemarie. And joined in with the rest of the life of the college.

We never did the Foundation Year. Later I was to wish we had.

The most important aspect of life at Emerson for me was social. I loved the dancing, the music, the House Meetings. I think Craig probably got more out of the course work. I particularly appreciated Adam Bittleston's current events contributions at House Meetings, and Francis's lectures on festivals. I learned a lot from you, Michael, in our work group in my eurythmy training year. I also remember having conversations about changes students wanted at school, and your openness to let them try it, even though some things had been tried before and not worked. There seemed to be a real active listening from the staff to students' needs which was welcome and impressive. In a way, because we were the cleaners, cooks, festival preparers, etc, we felt we were running the school with advice from our sage teachers and staff.

Anthony Kaye impressed me. When I was still 'fresh off the boat' (literally, as we arrived in Southampton on the QE II) Anthony stopped me in the narrow hallway in Pixton and said: 'How are you?'. Now, in my previous world (I had just graduated college in New Jersey) that was a throw-away line. No one expected an answer. But he stood there, looking intently and with interest at my face awaiting my answer. He actually wanted to know. Amazing!

Another time, towards the end of our biodynamic training when we were trying to figure out what to do next, Mr. Edmunds came down the same narrow hallway in Pixton. I flattened my tall self against the wall to let him pass. Instead of passing, he paused before me, pointed at my heart with his index finger and said: 'You should do eurythmy training'. I had never considered it. But later I found out that Molly had been talking about me in the Faculty Meetings. I slept on it and discovered it was right. You know how that impacted my life.

Craig stayed in biodynamic agriculture for 15 years. During that time we moved to Michael Hall and had two children. He could not find a position outside of a school where he could support a family in the US, so we stayed while he took the teacher training at Michael Hall with Brien Masters. He took a class where he could be mentored at Michael Hall for three years, then we finally returned to the

States after 16 years abroad! Instead of being little fishes in a big pond in Forest Row, all of a sudden we were trained and experienced Anthroposophists in a land with very few.

I started being very active in the local A Society, planning many festivals, teaching courses, leading study groups—all things we had attended before but not lead. Craig became College Chair after one year. He went on to be the lead teacher at a new Waldorf-inspired charter school.

Our children are 'lifers' i.e. they attended Waldorf Schools from pre-school through 12th grade. They went on to earn degrees at top schools and have successful careers in Mechanical Engineering and Economics.

We have much to be thankful for at Emerson. We learned Anthroposophy as well as life lessons. We have lifelong friends from that time. I remember Mr. Edmunds telling us at a House Meeting to 'look around. You see here the future leaders of Anthroposophical endeavours'. (That is not an exact quote). He was right. I know many of the leaders personally, at least of schools, training centers, etc. Many are from Emerson, even if they weren't there when we were.

Emerson wasn't for everyone. Some left. Some got ill. But for me, I blossomed like a bud in the sun.

One more little story, then I have to go sell jewellery (another job I have is making it): During our Agriculture Course, we were asked as a group to plan and lead the Easter Festival. We looked at each other and no one said anything. We had no idea what to do. So we started studying, reading, brainstorming, etc, and produced a fine festival on the day for the whole college. By the way, in our day, the whole college was huge. It included all the priest-training students, the social development people, the painting-training, sculpture (a four-year course then) 90 in the Foundation Year, etc. Anyway, along the way, I discovered I was a Christian, and had always believed in God. This was a huge thing. I was raised as an atheist and I was deep into Yoga at the time, but it came in a flash and was right. I have been a Christian ever since.

We are lucky to always have been able to work in our dream jobs. We found them at Emerson. I am grateful to my first eurythmy teacher, Molly, for opening that door for me. And grateful to have friends all over the country that shared that part of my life with me. Aloha, Anne

David Sloan (1971–2 and 1974–5)

During the 1971–2 Foundation Year, it looks as though some of the year took shape as follows:

—a general introduction to Anthroposophy, which included a description of biodynamics, plant ecology, and the planets from Herbert Koepf.

—Also early on that fall Francis gave a mind-blowing course on the three-fold human being.

—Adam Bittleston followed with a short course on the eight-fold path that expanded into an exploration of the 'I'.

—Ron Jarman presented imagination, inspiration and intuition and a course on the stars.

—John Davy offered a course on 'The Evolution of Man'.

—In a study group, we read *Theosophy*.

—Herbert Koepf also gave a course on 'The Evolution of the Earth'.

—Another course by Adam—'Evolution of Human Consciousness through Language'.

—I also remember doing speech with Graham Rickett, painting with Ann Stockton, projective geometry and Bothmer gymnastics with Olive Whicher, sculpture with John Wilkes, learning how to play the recorder, and doing eurythmy with Elizabeth Edmunds in the Hut. I believe John 'Chip' Wulsin and I were the only two students ever kicked out of one of her classes for sliding around the room in our socks, when she was trying to teach us how to move etherically!

In the spring, I recall spending a week with Van Houten and the NPI on social issues, and Dr. Mees also gave a short course on Karma and Illness. I believe Francis presented a course on the fundamentals of Waldorf education too.

Of course, when I look back on that first year, I am so utterly grateful that destiny worked its will. The karmic connections that intertwined then have continued for 40 years. There had been an American invasion that year—perhaps two-thirds of the 120 or so students—and the number of individuals I met that year with whom I still feel connected (even with those who have died) is astonishing—Michael Holdrege, James Pewtherer, John Wulsin, Peter von Breda, Curtis Wheeler, Frederick Whitcomb, Carol McCracken, Leslie Daugherty, Karin Bittleston, Keith McCrary, Bruce Mehrtens, and on and on. As young as I was (at 21 only Leslie was younger that year), and as overwhelming as the introduction to Anthroposophy was, it was also the turning point of my life. Every move I have made since bears the stamp of the people I met and the exposure to Rudolf Steiner's spiritual vision of humankind.

I left after one year because living in Forest Row had been a fairy tale of sorts, and I felt I needed to get some practical teaching experience before doing the Education Course. I returned two years later for the 1974–5 year. If my first year had been a turning point, this second year only deepened this feeling and the direction of my future. Of course, meeting Christine was the ultimate karmic connection, but there were others—Robert Koerber, the Daitz's, Kristin Waldrop (Ramsden), Christine and Paul Querido, Nina Sagall, Gale Langstroth, Joel Gordon, Robert Logsdon, Michael Connaughton, Chris and Debbie Day, Christopher Garvey, Alan Greene, et al.

In 1971–2, I had been a bit resistant to this new way of looking at the world, especially coming from a Jewish background and grappling with the immensity of the ideas leading to esoteric Christianity. By 1974–5, I had read a bit more of Steiner, and seemed readier inwardly to plunge into the work.

I wrote in my journal a couple of Francis's opening comments from the first course that fall—The Study of Man:

'We can only change the world in the measure that we change ourselves.'

'Where are the knights of today?'

'What gives you the right to be a teacher?'

Other Education Courses:
Eurythmy with Molly von Heider
Art with George Locher
Morning course on 'The Age of The Consciousness Soul'
Weekly Practice at Michael Hall
A morning course with John Davy on 'Psychology'
Lawrence Edwards—a short course on mathematics
Molly von Heider—a short course on 'The Etheric'
Margaret Shillan—an art course
Art History with Mr Mann
Jess Darrel—a short week on Religion

Norman Davidson—a week on maths
'The Mission of Biology' with Francis
A course on Language, and another on Geography taught be René Querido
Margaret Meyercourt—short course on the young child
Pedagogical conference with Francis and others
Eileen Hutchins—'The Mission of History and Literature'
Parsifal with Francis 'A study in the grounds of human idealism'
Curative Education with Stanley Price
Ron Jarman course on Teaching Science
Ursula Grahl on Fairy Tales
Frances Woolls on Chemistry
Arne Klingborg on Art
Drama workshop with Dawn Langman

A number of students were intensely interested in Shakespeare, so Francis met with us weekly in a non-curricular seminar. It led to an evening of Shakespeare scenes, and it certainly deepened our work with *King Lear* that spring. I played Gloucester, Paul Broadhead played Lear, Ronnie Goldberg was Albany, Jared Schuler played Edmund, Kristin Waldrop (Ramsden) played Regan, Christopher Garvey played Kent

Another great memory was the Mardi Gras evening in January, just before Christine and I went away to Cotswold Chine for our month-long practicum. Christine sang this burlesque number from 'Sweet Charity' called 'Don't Tell Mama', with a stony-faced chorus line of men in eurythmy veils moving solemnly behind her, performing 'm's' and 'f's' and 'ah's' as she belted out:

Mama, thinks I'm living in a convent in the southern part of France
Mama doesn't even have an inkling that I'm working in a nightclub in a pair of lacy pants
So please, sir, if you run into my mama, don't reveal my indiscretion, give a working girl a chance, etc.

I'm afraid I've rambled on way too long here, and have no idea whether these reminiscences have been even a little bit helpful. I do know that Emerson College represents the two most transformational years of my entire life, and that now at the advanced age of 61 I can look back with crystal clarity and see that those years were

really the 'eye of the needle' for me. Everything before 1971 was 'prologue', preparation for the challenge of meeting Anthroposophy and, even more importantly, the individuals in whom Anthroposophy lived so profoundly. Everything since that time has been an attempt to live in accordance with the ideals that I felt so strongly informed the work at Emerson.
David

Fritz Wessling (1981–2)

I was a Foundation Year student at Emerson College, from 1981 to 1982—a sort of gap-year, between my university training as an architect, and starting to work in my profession. What made me choose Emerson? Basically, the cosmopolitan atmosphere attracted me, the very social and artistic way I sensed Anthroposophy was lived and practised there, rather than just studied, as in many other places, according to my perception at the time. Being German by birth,(*1955) it had been clear from the start that I wanted to spend that year in another country, probably precisely for this reason ! Also I loved languages and meeting people from many different parts of the world, so Emerson seemed just right.

The Philosophy of Freedom held a special place. I was in Alistair MacDonald's study group, and am still deeply grateful for this experience to the present day. A friendship straddling an age difference of some 40 years developed quickly; we gravitated towards one another in many tea breaks, and had splendid conversations. Even now, decades after his passing, I often experience his kind, lucid and encouraging spirit as being close. One of the key qualities I deeply appreciated at Emerson was the fact that teachers met students always at eye level, never up to down. And Alistair was a master in this, treating me, the greenhorn in Anthroposophy, as a young colleague ... My course group leaders were Myra MacDonald and Paul Matthews. Doris Meeks was my Eurythmy teacher, and with Dawn Langman I did speech. During first term we went through several arts and crafts workshops. I took part in the Christmas plays (an adaption of the Coventry plays written by Francis Edmunds). In the King's play, I remember John Davy playing the red and myself the black devil. During second term, I did painting with Anne Stockton, and during third term, sculpture with

Rudolf Kaesbach. Especially this deepening artistic work with Anne and Rudolf has been nourishment for my soul ever since. I also went to William Mann's Art History classes one evening a week, and in third term, I attended a study group with him about the Manifestations of Karma.

Looking back, it is no exaggeration to say that this year at Emerson has been at the core of everything important I have endeavored to do in my life ever since. A kind of basis for anything fruitful I set out to do later on in life. How fortunate I was ! The expectations I brought when I came to Emerson were all met or exceeded, and perhaps the most precious thing was that people there lived what they were teaching, in their daily lives with us, students. I definitely experienced the Emerson College approach to Anthroposophy as my own. Today's spirituality as social art, the deep respect for each human being, the transformative power of the arts, a relation to the spirit world based entirely on individual human freedom—these and many more qualities and virtues I was able to witness and take in. And last but not least, the sense of humour that was very much present in the mood of the place. A good laugh can help put things into perspective. Anthroposophy can and should be fun in certain moments. Emerson College—a great example for everybody!
São Romão, Portugal, May 1st, 2011

Holly Johnson (1980–2)

16 May 2011

Dear Michael,
It is with pleasure that I put down some words about my Emerson Experience. It was a turning point in my life that brought me to my true profession and passion after many years of 'searching' for what my purpose was. Take what you like, I will be writing this as I recall those two marvelous years.

My Foundation Year (1980) is vague as I think I was absorbing what my Waldorf Education had given me. I never knew who Rudolf Steiner was. At Emerson I was hearing words like Spiritual Freedom, Occult Science, and Theosophy! 'What kind of school is this?' Who, What, Where???I remember John Davy giving the opening for the morning lessons with humour and a joyous smiling face.

He was always seen on campus greeting us, active in the Study Groups and ready to delve into 'the deeper questions'. John Meeks gave a course on Parsifal, which was way over my head. Olive Whicher on Botany, John Wilkes on Flowforms and then Biodynamics and the Rural Development with Mr. Koepf who's wife, Ursula, took me on as a project in healing my voice doing Verbeck Singing. I know you were the Bursar and did a talk on the Threefold Social Order. My Study Group was lead by John Meeks; I became engrossed in *The Philosophy of Freedom*, having concepts that were planted early in my life come to my understanding as we all grappled with the New Thought.

I remember seeing Francis Edmunds 'from a distance' as I was not sure how to approach this man who I had so much admiration for.

I do remember Molly quite well because she was encouraging me to participate in Eurythmy and I was insistent that after 12 years of causing trouble for Miss Puderoran (Eurythmy teacher at Highland Hall) there was no way I was entering the Eurythmy Hall. This went on for the entire year. Finally as I entered my Teachers Training Year she convinced me to 'Just watch'. I did and fell in love with it!!!

To this day I thank Molly for helping me embrace Eurythmy.

I loved all the Festivals. Especially the International Evening where we came together in our Country Groups to give a taste of who we are. My group did a Square Dance and passed out Popcorn as if in a Baseball Park.

Mayfair was the best! The gum boots lined up around the circle to step into as we sloshed around the maypole.

Rural Development Garden was awe inspiring and the place I went to be quiet. The kitchen, oh the kitchen. I loved helping there and gained quite a bit of weight too! And then . . .

I met the woman who was always there behind me, never obvious but always there when I was about to burst into tears. Roswitha! My mentor, guide, angel.

As she led me into the Batik Room I found my solace, my passion, my comfort, and my dear Batik partner Dorit Summerfield. The two of us 'lived in the Batikery'. Every spare minute we were there. Through lunch and dinner we were there. Into the night we were there. I made a lampshade as a gift to Emerson which was in the lobby by your office . . . whatever happened to it? We gave a Batik Art Show. *Cymbeline* our Shakespeare Play was done in Batik!

Emerson College gave me back what I lost when I was no longer a Waldorf Student.

It gave me DIRECTION and PASSION for Waldorf Education! It answered why I was always SEARCHING, QUESTIONING; as I love to explore and meet and see. It gave me REASON to BE. It quenched my thirst AND opened my eyes for SPIRITUAL KNOWLEDGE. It allowed me to live in COMMUNITY with other cultures, a lifestyle I still search for and hope to find again.

Emerson College helped me to become a CONFIDENT WALDORF TEACHER, A CREATIVE AND IMAGINATIVE WOMAN.

Thank you!
HOLLY JOHNSON

P.S. After Graduation I went to Camphill Le Beal in France and Camphill Beannachar in Scotland. Class and Handwork Teacher at Summerfield Waldorf School, Santa Rosa Ca. Handwork teacher (thank you Roswitha) at Journey Charter School, Aliso Viejo Ca. ESL teacher in China and now unemployed and looking for my next step!

You asked which speakers/teachers we had.
1st: Evolution of Man—John Davy, Sept 19, 1980. I have all my notes. The very last writing I have says 'SPIRITUALITY IS THE A-HA OF LIFE'.
2nd: Projective Geometry—Olive Wicher
3rd: Evolution of Drama and Poetry—Paul Matthews and Dawn Langman
4th: Mathematics—Ron Jarman, so far my favourite spokesman!
5th: Study of Man—William Mann (isn't that Roswitha's dad?) Nov 24, 1980
6th: Psychology—Social Development Centre, Tijno Voors, Christopher Shaefer, Hester Goodwin
7th: Science and Technology—John Davy, Jan 26, 1981. This lecture touched on the world of computers ... wow! For me they didn't enter into my life for another 10 years
8th: Karma-Destiny—Adam Bittleston
9th: Parsifal ... guess I didn't like this class as I didn't write down the lecture's name, and my notes are full of doodles! Actually Form Drawings, thank you Roswitha
10th: Basic Attitudes—Social Dev Centre

11th: Medicine—Dr. Twentyman, May 4, 1981
12th: Darkness and Light—Michael Wilson
13th: Development of Architecture ... no name but I have wonderful drawings, or doodles ... hum...

With love and fondness,
Holly Johnson

Katherine Christine (1972–5)

Hello Michael,
Well, yes as Elizabeth once said we were FAMOUS, the first group of eurythmists.

All the students came out of a course at Emerson, mostly out of the Foundation Year. We arrived together.

...I have often thought about what happened in those years and what was able to happen because of Emerson.

I also think that we planned and organized this well before we were born.

Wherever could one arrive, not know the slightest thing about Eurythmy, do it in the Foundation Year, see it as one's life's goal and then be able to start something on home ground so to speak and then carry on somewhere else?

Of course it was a unique and pioneer situation and that's what made it so very Emerson. We could all be born thousands of miles apart on different sides of the world, develop what we needed for our own individual destinies and then unite for a short but very important time in order to carry our impulses into the world. This was the very 'soil' of Emerson at that time, a place for meeting up to do what we had set out for. I don't blame John Davy for being so against it at the beginning. He had his loyalties to Marguerite and wanted to support her School. But for us this was so to speak something that we had already planned a long time ago.

Not everybody was able to see that.

I once had a dream about the college. It stood on a hill, as it does and leading from the building was a beautiful bridge. Many people were there and that picture has remained with me. Emerson as the bridge from the spiritual world before birth and then the place where you can come, meet the right people and then carry on. Take my life for example. Where in God's name (or in God's Africa) could I have found Eurythmy? Where would I have gone? There was really only this possibility. Where and how would I have found my teachers, first Elizabeth then Molly von Heider who was the bridge to Klink.

Of course it was a good initiative. We were also prepared to take the risk. We trained in the first years without recognition from Dornach. That was a risk and it turned out to be a good thing. We all became eurythmists and that is what counts in the end.

I have many other thoughts about Emerson and think very often about it as well. I recently looked at some group photos and realized that one carries these people within oneself.

Love Katherine

Keith McCrary (1971–3 (PLUS))

It was in the winter of 1971. The place was San Francisco. I was 35 years old. I was working as a freelance artist—a caricature street artist at Fisherman's Wharf, the city's main tourist attraction. Before that, for three years I had been the pastor of the First Methodist Church of San Francisco. I had been married for 10 years with three great children—and then divorced. Oops! That wasn't supposed to happen.

This was the era of hippies and my housemate at the time certainly qualified by the looks of him. This was a time of radical experimentation. Talk of revolution was in the air. In spite of Martin Luther King's assassination, the Civil Rights Movement was still very much alive. The Vietnam War was winding down. Free Schools were popping up in many places, especially on the West Coast. Many felt something new was just around the corner.

In this context I was urged to attend a lecture by L. Francis Edmunds, who was touring the U.S. to recruit students for Emerson College. As I was looking to return to teaching, one of my former parishioners, Ruth Jung, asked me one day if I had ever heard of Rudolf Steiner. It turned out her best friend was an Anthroposophist, and they thought I should become a Waldorf teacher.

It so happened I had heard of Rudolf Steiner and Waldorf Education in the early '60s. In my third year as a high school history and English teacher I had come across the young Sacramento Waldorf School. It was then two years old. I had even attended a weeklong conference at Highland Hall in the Los Angeles area in the summer of 1961.

So there I was 10 years later listening to this man with a delightful English accent. He was in his late 60s at that time. He caught my attention with two thoughts. 'Unless your life is a saga, you're merely existing!' I could relate, totally. My life was definitely a saga, and I have only given you a glimpse of the craziness of my life in the Bay Area from 1962 on.

However, the most enticing thing Francis had to say that evening was as follows: 'Waldorf education is not a system. It is a movement. If you would like to help shape this movement, come along and join us.'

In the months that followed a flurry of events took place. I arranged to rent Jeanne Bailey's house, Chequer Farm, on Highgate Road near Michael Hall in Forest Row. Lynette Mann and I were married in a half-hippie wedding in a San Francisco public park near the ocean. We sold most all of our belongings, including two cars. I borrowed $9000 from a wealthy heiress friend, and with Lynette's son from her previous marriage, we flew off to London and then on to Sussex by early August. And the saga continued.

My first impressions of Emerson College included the great space in front of Pixton House and throwing a Frisbee with Dave Alsop. He and his wife, Marianne, would become lifelong friends. Later Marianne and Lynette became business partners for 14 years. They owned a toy and bookstore called The Ark in Fair Oaks, CA. Other long-term friendships began that year with John Wulsin, Peter van Breda, and Van James to name a few.

All of the people working with the college were special: the Horsfalls, the cook—Anthony Kaye, the Tablehurst Farm manager, Katherine Castelliz, elderly Lionel in the book bindery, and the ladies in the library and the secretaries in the office.

All of the teachers and other community members were exceptional people: Francis and of course his amazing wife, Elizabeth Edmunds, John and Gudrun Davy, Herbert and Ursula Koepf, Anne Stockton, Olive Whicher, Julian Pook, Graham Rickett, Hagen Biesantz, Dr. Laine Mees, 'Mookie' Mann, Rudy Lissau, Margaret Meyercourt, Eileen Hutchins, Ron Jarman, John Wilkes, Cecil Harwood, Roswitha and Michael Spence, among others. Though much could be said about each of these people, perhaps the most influential person for me was Adam Bittleston.

Early in my first year Adam introduced the season of Michaelmas with a memorable statement: 'No one has escaped from breathing the breath of the dragon.' The way in which he said it brought seriousness to the event and made it clear that he knew what he was talking about. Adam also lectured on the Eight-Fold Path in a way that was fresh, creative and provocative. I have often referred to my notes when considering the subject and its relationship to the chakra of the throat. I also attended his weekly Star Course. He made the zodiac come alive.

An experience I had during one of Elizabeth Edmunds's Eurythmy classes was of some significance in my life. Because of previous involvement with modern dance, I felt very open to and appreciative of Eurythmy. Then one day in the middle of class, I began to notice diaphanous colours around my classmates. It was the first time I had experienced seeing auras. Afterward I told Elizabeth. She beamed and grabbed my hand and said quietly but enthusiastically, 'Oh my! Oh my!' It made me aware of how powerful Eurythmy is with regard to the expansion of human consciousness.

I had come to Emerson as an enquirer. I asked all sorts of questions about Rudolf Steiner, his philosophy, his life and work. I had spent the year pursuing these questions when a major insight occurred to me.

It was June of 1972. I was riding a train into London. I was reading what was then called *Occult Science*, when three words came to me: 'Spirit precedes matter.' Later I would read similar phrasing in Steiner's writing. I also realized these words expressed a parallel thought that is found in the prologue to John's gospel. This had long been a daily mantram for my meditative life: 'In the beginning was the Word and the Word became flesh full of grace and truth . . .' It became clear there was no major conflict between the traditional Christian experience of the truth of unconditional love (grace) and what Anthroposophy was pointing to. In fact, Anthroposophy deepens this central reality.

Having been a Class Teacher for 29 years and increasingly involved in Adult Waldorf Education (AWE) for these past several years, I am especially appreciative that Rudolf Steiner had the foresight to bring into being a practical way of expressing this amazing grace for humankind.

Forty years ago Francis Edmunds invited me to come along and help shape the movement called Waldorf. According to some of the feedback of my former students, it seems I have continued the stream of caring that goes along with being a Waldorf teacher. If I have contributed anything significant to the movement perhaps it has been humour. The adage that angels know how to fly because they take themselves lightly still resonates with me.

Mary Lee Plumb-Mentjes (1960–70)

I attended the Foundation Year in 1969–1970.

I turned 20 that fall. Piet (now passed on) and Heather Ross and I were the three youngest. John Turner and Violet Bursey may have been the oldest in that year. It was really wonderful the full span of ages and nationalities of my year. It's funny that I don't remember particulars about the incredible morning courses and speakers. For one of the few times in my life I took very few notes; I felt that everything went straight into my heart and served truly as a renewing wellspring for my idealism. In perhaps the only interview I had with Mr. Edmunds he expressed concern that perhaps I had had experiences in the Civil Rights Movement in America (jailed for civil disobedience in Washington, D.C. and working a summer in rural Mississippi), which actually was invigorating, but more particularly working in the Haight Ashbury in San Francisco as a co-worker in a halfway house for a drug treatment centre where there were heroin addicts and worse, young teens who had experience with uppers and downers that had already put them in hospital; they came out like old people with no spark left. It was a time where the encounter groups move each participant to a least common denominator. Co-workers weren't to rely on any title/position for separation; we shared the same bedrooms. As a young, untried idealist I was a sitting duck. Right before I left for Emerson, I came to the point where I felt 'at least I have this, this small pile in front of me, being like a miser'. When I went to Emerson (which was just because my father had already paid the deposit), I felt this incredible affirmation that 'there is more; I knew there was/is'. It was like going through a crossing point and coming out the other side at Emerson.

At the time my understanding was that Mr. Edmunds wanted people with life experience. Looking back I can see his point because I have little cognitive memory of the courses, but I still feel that the period right before I went to Emerson was the lowest point of my life and that Emerson quickened the flame of the best part of me and that I have not forgotten. I loved the morning verse that was said in the common room: 'We will to work, letting flow through our work what... And as life-bodily wills to become man in us.' The year before mine I heard that some students did not want to do kitchen work or work on the farm; they just wanted to have time to study. I couldn't believe that anyone could have that attitude. I loved vegetable preparation in the morning with Anthony. We would show each other the beautiful forms seen in the cut vegetables. I loved doing scullery with Jon Godber singing opera and John Turner. I loved Thursday afternoons when we worked on the farm. I wrote poems about the setting sun and the colours of the fall cabbage-leaves with the waning light. We gathered for a poetry group meeting in an old caravan once or twice. I remember Misha (Michael) Howard taking part. I remember that I demonstrated the same planning qualities I showed with the start of our local Waldorf school; I remembered to bring toilet paper. I remember my best birthday ever when I could sit in a corner at Rachel Clayfield's (later Shepherd) and Anne Stockton's and enjoy the lovely candlelight; it was mainly for Rachel's birthday, but I had a crown of marigolds. I was so fond of Amalia Torres (from Colombia) who lived there too; I think Elizabeth Edmunds wondered at our differences; for Amalia it was as though I was her connection to earthly things like bread and jam. I am embarrassed how I made a crude long purple skirt like Amalia's to wear. I became exhausted by all of the people and took a rest after lunch in a little room upstairs that I think Helen O'Reilly found for me. When I would lie there I would dream/imagine what I could make, generally from things I found in nature, for each person's birthday. My room on Chapel Lane was truly like a squirrel's nest. I'd like to refind the person who wrote poems and created from nature (I still am known as someone who remembers people's birthdays). I remember Jeremy sitting in one of the big comfortable chairs in the common room at the close of day, and once on an evening walk through the farm.

15
Staff Arrangements and Salaries

When I joined Emerson I stepped into a work and a way of life that was very different from everything I had become accustomed to before. I found myself amongst a group of people who accepted as fact a spiritual reality that was there behind the everyday world in which we lived and worked. But they did this, in the main, in a way that was entirely devoid of sentimentality, dogma or undue emotion. It was not a belief based on religious teaching but something that made sense of life; that gave meaning and purpose to all that we were involved in.

As I explained in chapter 4, when Francis Edmunds invited me to join the college he worked in a way that clearly separated the work a person did from the salary he was given—the salary was not money in exchange for work. I found myself feeling very much at home in such a way of thinking. Clearly in my mind this was work I wanted to do, and to do it for its own sake. The salary freed me to do it. In this and in much else of a similar nature to which I was led, not only by Francis Edmunds but also by Lionel Elin and others, I was prompted to look again at all my conventional understanding of money, of legal arrangements, administrative procedures, and social forms.

Lionel Elin gave me from his own library an old copy of Rudolf Steiner's lectures published as *World Economy*, with which I immediately experienced a strong connection. Then later he gave me other books on the threefold social order. In the early 1970s I began running study groups on the 'threefold social order', and on *World Economy*.* Later I was also asked to give lectures to the Foundation Year and the Agricultural Courses. Looking back I am always surprised at the enthusiasm of the students as I was certainly no expert, I too was learning. But the questions they brought and the discussions that followed were enormously important in helping me develop my understanding of the subject—I have a strong belief that I actually learned more than they did.

Clearly, if Emerson was to be true to itself and to the needs of the students who came, then the administrative and financial arrangements we came to had to be formed out of those spiritual truths on which the

* Rudolf Steiner, *World Economy* (Rudolf Steiner Press, 1972).

college was founded. Otherwise there would be a lie embedded in the very fabric of the college. I felt it particularly important that a person, whether a student or someone from the world at large, coming into the office met there, consciously or unconsciously, the same truths that the students met in the classrooms and experienced in the festivals. This was especially important in the way we dealt with money and legal matters. This could be a real challenge. We were not always able to achieve it but that the effort was made was itself important. The college had to strive always to be true within itself.

Just as students came in order to fulfil a need they experienced within the depths of their souls, so also those who came as staff came because within their own soul's depths they felt a need to join in this community of work. Their own lives' path had led them to it.

If this was true, and I have no doubt about it being true of the great majority of the staff even if many were not fully conscious of it, would it be true to them and to the spiritual realities on which the college was founded, to put a monetary value on their work and pay them according to that value, to purchase their labour? This was not the usual situation of an employer employing people to do certain work. The people who came did so because of the particular nature of the work and the community of life in the college. Those who rightfully found their way to the college recognized, consciously or unconsciously, that their karma had led them to it. The work they came to was the work that would bring, at least for a certain period of their life, fulfilment and purpose to their lives.

In law the college could quite properly be seen as a body corporate, a being in itself, but spiritually it was a group of free human beings who, out of their individual destinies and intentions had come together to carry a common work in community, or association. We did not create predetermined job descriptions which we then looked for someone to fill, but rather looked for someone who out of his own biography and life's impulses seemed to be the person to enter into or take on a particular area of work. This deeper relationship between the individual and the organization was fundamental to Emerson College and informed much of the contractual arrangements between the two parties. We had, of course, to find ways of fulfilling the requirements of the State and at the same time to be true to the Spiritual World.

There was something else that needed to be recognized and accepted by those committing themselves to the work. The college was founded to serve individuals who had set out on a search for a path to the Spirit. If we were to make it possible for these, mostly young, people for whom it was created, to actually come to the college, then we had to find a balance between the needs of the staff and the financial possibilities of those students. As the situation was at that time both in the college and in the world at large there was no way that the college could fulfil its purpose if it tried to employ the number of staff, pay the sort of salaries and create the standard of facilities usual for such institutions. It is certainly true that for the first 25 or 30 years the great majority of staff worked longer hours and received less money than was normal in the world at large, or even in many other anthroposophical institutions. Added to this was the fact that students spent more time in contact with a teacher, or in a learning situation, and benefited from a richer cultural social life than they could expect almost anywhere else.

This is not the place to discuss the threefold nature of social life except to say that the work of the college came first and foremost within the cultural sphere of that life. What the student paid as tuition fee and the teacher received as salary can only be truly understood when considered as gift or more properly as contribution rather than as purchase and sale. Other supportive areas of activity such as cooking, maintenance, board and lodging, though really economic in nature were generally treated as within the overall cultural nature of the college.

As explained above, when someone came to work at the college, it was the work itself that was important and gave him or her a sense of fulfilment in life. This was particularly true, but not only so, for teachers; this was their lives' work, even if only until their life took them on to other work elsewhere. The money a person was given bore no relationship to the work he did, but to his needs. If one sets out to move away from the usual basis of buying a person's work or labour, then one cannot calculate what one pays him on the basis of that work. As soon as one arrives at a salary in any way conditioned by a person's qualifications, experience, type of work, or the actual number of hours worked, then one is thinking in terms of the commodity value of the work and paying according to that value—one is paying for the work, buying an integral part of that other person. In such a relationship the person employed is not a free human being; something of him is sold, his labour belongs to another. At Emerson the importance of freedom was fundamental. For the individual to be free the work and the calculation of salary had to be kept completely separate.

There was of course a certain relationship between work and pay in that only those who made a full-time commitment could expect to have their needs met fully. But this full commitment was not defined in terms of hours, some people are simply not able to work at the same intensity or for as long as others. A person who took on responsibility for a certain work recognized by the college as within that person's capacity would be given a salary calculated solely on his needs to the extent that that work was recognized as a full-time commitment.

Because each person experienced his work as entirely separated from his pay, as something he did for its own sake, each came to a freer sense of doing the work out of impulses arising within him or herself. Many found this gave them a remarkable uplifting experience. Due to the fact that it was one's own work each developed a sense of responsibility for that work and for the work of the college as a whole. Though for legal purposes everyone was an employee, in reality each experienced the work as his own. Because of this, individuals were much more flexible and, with fewer emotional blockages, were able on occasion to adjust their salary needs downwards when this became necessary as the college went through a period of financial difficulties. So too they would take on extra work when that was needed. The circle of staff, or colleagues as we thought of ourselves, experienced it as their college, not themselves as employees doing what they were paid to do. There were no salary scales or contracted hours of work. Nor were there any contracts of employment beyond that required by law; nor job descriptions laying down details of the work to be done.

Just as every person who came to work at the college was individual and different from anyone else, so were the paths by which they came, and the procedures through which they were accepted, different and particular to them. But generally what follows is what happened. A person's proposed involvement would first be discussed in a personal conversation. At the beginning this would have been with Francis Edmunds, later with a small group. The group would probably consist of two or three members of the Council plus at least one member of staff from the area of work the prospective new member would be coming to join. For example if he was to join the kitchen staff, then someone from the kitchen would be involved, or if to teach art then an art teacher. I would also normally be included, at least when they came to discuss financial and other such arrangements. The question of their financial needs and what the college could contribute generally came after both sides had agreed the wish for him or her to join the staff of the college.

Once I had settled into my work and had come to some understanding of my task and its nature I always tried to explain to anyone joining the staff circle the way the college was organized and the financial implications of working at the college. Due to the limited financial circumstances of many of the sort of students we set out to work with we could not pay the sort of salaries or give the security that would normally be expected elsewhere. For the foreseeable future we could not provide for staff to buy their own houses nor to retire with a comfortable pension. They were coming to do this work because this was the work they themselves chose and wished to do. It was important that they recognized that it was their decision to join the college and this should be made in full consciousness of the step they were taking. The college would do its best to meet their needs, if necessary into retirement and beyond, but life did not make it possible to give any honest guarantees.

It was only after arrangements had been verbally agreed that details would be confirmed in writing, though at the beginning even this was not always done.

Salaries

The intention was to pay people a regular salary calculated according to each individual's needs. This did not mean we paid whatever a person needed or wanted; we were probably never in the position to do that. The aim was to pay everyone an equal proportion of their needs. How we assessed 'needs' was often discussed but never definitely established. Just as every human being is unique and individual so each has different needs particular to him or her. If an organization, in this age of the consciousness soul, seriously recognizes this, it cannot in all honesty treat one person as having the same or equal needs as another. Some people, for example, actually need to feel well-dressed while others are comfortable in their old clothes or in jeans; some have a real fear of the uncertainty of the future, while others have a confidence in their own destiny. These feelings are realities, they are not right or wrong, they are part of each of us; something we have to work out for ourselves. To be faithful to the spiritual truths on which the college was founded and continued to teach we could not say to a person that he 'should' be different than he was, or have different needs than he did have. Whereas conventional salary structures are based on the commodity value of a person's labour or skills, and most needs-based salary schemes generally treat people as all the same, at Emerson we tried to arrange salaries according to the individual nature of each person. If true community is to arise, each member needs to accept, and help provide for, other's particular individual problems and needs.

In actual practice, as I have previously explained, because everyone who joined the college came to experience themselves as an equal member of, and responsible for, the college as a whole, they also came to a sense of a common level of need or standard of living. A new person joining would sometimes need a certain time to develop this sense. I remember one couple in particular who started with unusually high but for them real needs and over each of the next two years they themselves asked for an actual reduction in salary, despite inflation.

As I have already indicated, the college was never in a position to pay the sort of salaries that would enable people to buy their own houses and retire on a good pension. This was something we all had to recognize and accept as a necessary part of our commitment to working with those who came as students to the college. Not everyone found it easy. In fact for many of us it was something we had to struggle with. It was often a real challenge to actually take into our will forces what we had come to understand as destiny, karma, and reincarnation. When faced with questions of money a person's convictions can come under real challenge. I remember Coen van Houten once saying that 'In this Michaelic age we have to learn to develop the courage to face the future that we ourselves have prepared for ourselves.' This thought was something that I always found enormously helpful. I do believe that something of this struggle was experienced in the spiritual environment of Emerson by many people, particularly the students who spoke of Emerson as a special place.

In the early years the college provided a minimum cash salary and where possible it itself found housing, including all services. There was an agreed policy that there should be staff living on campus. This was not primarily because it was cheaper for the college, but because it was important for the life of the students that staff did not all disappear at the end of the working day but were there as part of the life of the community, particularly at weekends. The Edmunds themselves, the Wilkes and Spence families with their children, the Koepfs, Molly von Heider, Ilse Brice, Dana Prager, and others all lived on campus. Others lived in houses we acquired in the village. There were also quite a number who already owned their houses in the vicinity before joining the college. Of these, some were retired people who were very committed to the college and active in different ways, generally in part-time teaching, most of whom did not want any financial support.

Where the college housed a member of staff, the intention was that this should be treated as their home where they would have a right to live as long as they continued to work at the college and if necessary into retirement. This, of course, was dependant on their having put a substantial part of their lives' work into the college. But it meant also that when they died the house came back to the college rather than to their descendants. Instead of paying salaries that allowed them, after tax, to buy their own houses, the college itself built housing on campus, or purchased them in the village. In this way the college over the years built up a valuable collection of houses. The custom accepted by the Inland Revenue in Britain at that time allowed educational establishments to house their staff without the staff having to pay tax on the benefit. I personally checked this with the tax authorities. It is unlikely that this would be possible today. This arrangement was of enormous financial benefit to the college and, I do believe, more than offset the cost to the college of continuing to house the few members who stayed on after retirement.

Salaries were reviewed each year. On the Council we would look at the likely financial situation of the college for the coming year particularly in the light of expected circumstances in the wider world. We would look at such factors as any possible increase or decrease in student and staff numbers and therefore of income and expenditure for the year ahead, and at possible changes in inflation, exchange rates and cost of living. From this we would then come to a recommendation of a salary increase, or decrease, for the coming year. This would then be explained and discussed at a Staff Meeting. The figure agreed as recommendation was really a guideline. Members of staff were then asked to review their own individual situations, and put, in writing or verbally, to a member of the salary committee, the salary they would need for the coming year. If they did not make any specific request they would be paid the recommended increase. We always worked on a net figure, that is, the amount they would receive after tax, National Insurance and any other such deductions. It was always emphasized that if circumstances changed during the year they could always approach any member of the salary group for an additional increase or lump sum.

If someone asked for what we felt on the salary committee to be an unexpected amount one of us would talk to that person. In actual practice over the years we approached more people because we felt they were not looking after their own needs sufficiently and were asking too little, than because we felt a person was asking more than seemed reasonable. We did not all know what each received as salary. While I was bursar there were three occasions when we discussed in the staff circle whether we wanted to continue with the present salary system or change to some other, and also whether we should all know what everyone received. On each occasion, with few reservations the decision was to continue as at present, though sometimes with a few minor alterations, usually to the structure or role of the salary committee. With regard to knowing or not knowing what each was paid; John Davy put it very well on one occasion. He pointed to the fact that if he knew what each was paid but did not know all their inner and outer circumstances of the person, their life problems, and biographical background, he could not bring an objective judgement to the knowledge. The danger then was that it became an emotional judgement and this could have a damaging effect on personal relationships and the life of the community. He said he joined the college in order to work with students; he could not also go into all the life details of all his colleagues. That should be left to a few people in whom we all had confidence. The great majority of the staff agreed with this.

At salary discussion meetings I often reminded colleagues that in reality it was not the college which paid our salaries but our students. The college had little other income. Whatever we decided to pay ourselves would have a direct effect on the fees and so could make it more difficult, or even impossible, for some students for whom the college was created to come. These students did not come to the college by chance or accident but found their way through their karma. Most would have actual karmic connections to one or other of us. In the deepest sense these were, for the present, 'our' students.

During the early years there were a large number of older people who made very important contributions to the life of the college. Students enormously valued what they gave of their wisdom, wisdom gained through lives committed to and active in anthroposophy. Some lived locally while others were full-time or visiting staff housed by the college. They loved to work with the students, wishing only to give what they could. Many of them had passed or were approaching retirement age and asked for little or no salary or other financial support. Some, committed to a full-time programme, did need housing and some financial support, but they lived substantially on their pensions or other savings and so could be said to give far out of proportion to what they received. Though it is impossible to list them all I feel I should mention here people like Lionel and Marcia Elin, Alistair and Myra Macdonald, Conrad Saxon-Snell, William Mann, Violet Bursey, Olive Whicher, Barbara Saunders-Davies, Adam Bittleston, Herbert and Ursula Koepf, Ilse Brice, Gerda Hillman, Anne Stockton, Gisela Bittleston, Ann Gooding, and Katherine Castelliz.

What all these and many others gave to the students of their lives' experience and wisdom was of incalculable importance. That they could give so much with so little financial cost to the college enabled the college not only to keep the fees down, but it meant that more resources could be used for the development of the college with the essential new buildings and infrastructure required for the growing work. But, more importantly, what so many freely gave out of love for the students and their commitment to the work of the spirit could be experienced in the etheric life of the college long after they themselves had passed on, even to this day. This, of course, was also true of those who gave in other ways and of all those young people who came and gave of their work during the holidays.

* * *

In the early days there was no talk of retirement. Francis was already in his 60s when he founded the college and 66 years old when the college moved to Pixton. The idea that at a predetermined age one retired, stopped doing the work that gave meaning and purpose to life, suddenly letting go of the responsibilities and commitments that one had previously carried, seemed extraordinary and unreal. Age should bring a slowing down, or a giving up of some work and taking on other more appropriate to old age. In the early pioneer-time we did not immediately take up the question of pensions. The assumption was that, like so many of the older contributors, we would continue to work into old age, just slowing down. Life had meaning and purpose and this did not suddenly end at an arbitrary age of 60 or 65. When we came to set up pension arrangements, this was thought of in the way of giving some security against the unpredictability of old age, but more in the sense that it would help the college to continue to support us as our work slowed down.

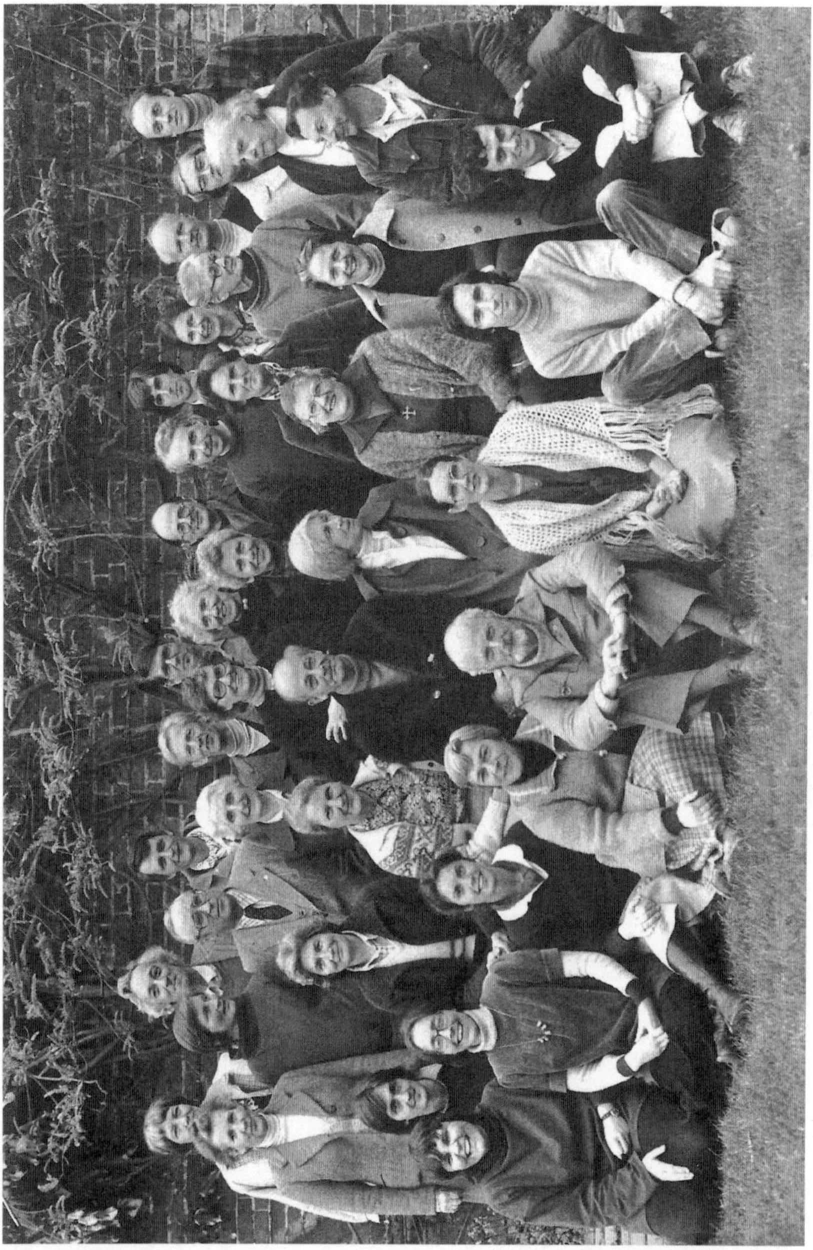

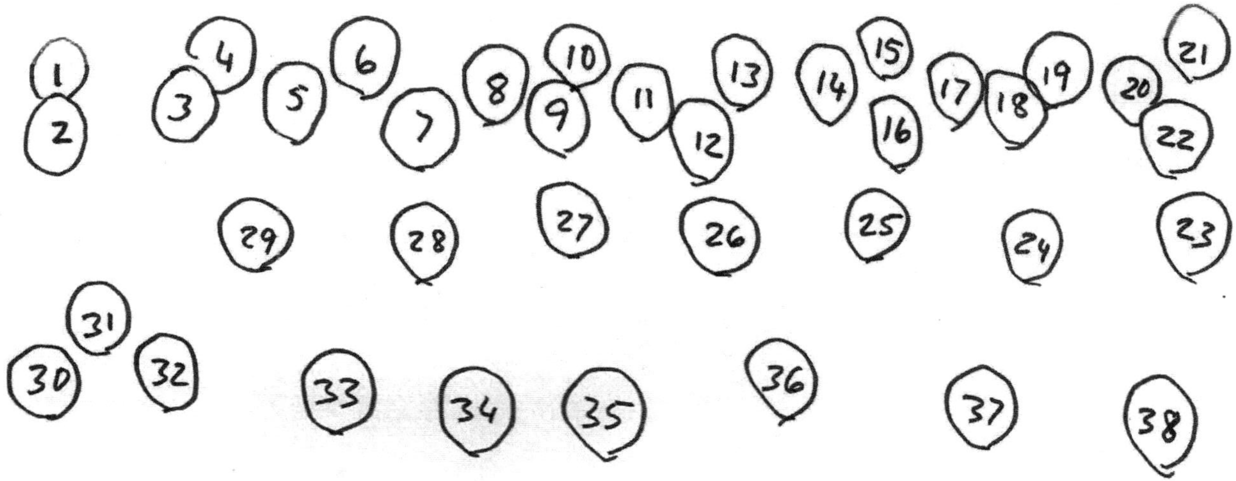

Staff, mid-1970s (see diagram): 1. Djobs van Houten, 2. Ilse Brice, 3. Annemarie Vinkhuyzen, 4. Ron Jarman, 5. Herbert Koepf, 6. Tijno Voors, 7. Olive Whicher, 8. Conrad Saxon-Snell, 9. Gudrun Davy, 10. John Davy, 11. Molly von Heider, 12. Eva Kulka, 13. Peter Horsfall, 14. Julian Pook, 15. John Meeks, 16. Anne Brocklebank, 17. Doris Meeks, 18. Barbara Saunders-Davies, 19. Michael Spence, 20. Violet Eursey, 21. Bill Day, 22. Gerda Hillman, 23. Mark Feedman, 24. Roswitha Spence, 25. Dana Prager, 26. Elizabeth Edmunds, 27. Leen Mees, 28. Anne Stockton, 29. Myra Macdonald, 30. Dawn Langman, 31. Patrick Stolfo, 32. Brenda Ratcliffe, 33. Lesley Cox, 34. Ursula Koepf, 35. Alistair Macdonald, 36. Irene Bruntsch, 37. Don Ratcliffe, 38. Paul Matthews

16
Board, Lodging, and Tuition Fees

Marjorie Theyer (1965–7) wrote:

> *It was Francis who brought me to the college and found me the job at Nutley when I didn't have any money. I literally bumped into him on New Year's day during a snow storm!!! He gave me tea in the wooden huts up on the Eastbourne Rd and then I wanted to go to Emerson . . . he then spent months trying to dissuade me. In the spring Mary Rose, Gay and I went to a weekend at Peredur and then I was more determined to go!!! So in the end, he said he would find me a job that would give me a roof over my head and good food and pocket money and I could pay him back when I had some money so that another student could then come to Emerson because it didn't matter to him whether he taught 20 or 21 people!!! I did pay him back each term. I was teaching and every time he wrote me a personal note of thanks!!! Such was the man.*

Before going into student fees themselves there is something I should explain.

One of the primary tasks of the Foundation Year was to help students on to their path of inner development and an awakening to the spirit within them. But this is a lonely path, a journey each has to do for himself. No one can do it for another, or accompany him in his struggle. Another can point the way, tell him what he will meet on his path, but the actual inner journey and all that is involved in it an individual can only do for himself alone. All inner striving and searching for knowledge and understanding are activities arising out of the needs of the human ego. They are by that fact lonely and egoistic activities. They cannot be other. This is the nature of the cultural sphere of human community. Over against this, in the social life of the community, there must be that which provides a balance; that provides a community of human warmth and support around this lonely path. The individual cannot provide this for himself. In the wider human community the polarity to the cultural life is, or should be, the economic productive activity of the community. A study of this economic productive sphere will show that the activity itself quite practically calls for mutuality or brotherhood, for each providing, not for himself, but for others. This is not a matter of dogma, or 'because

Rudolf Steiner said so'. It is a fact clearly discernible to anyone who takes the time and determination to look deeply into the matter.

At Emerson something of this was provided in the way we attempted to work with money, particularly with student fees. In the college community we tried to move away from the prevailing tendency of the domination of money where everything has a cost and must be charged and paid for, where everyone pays for what they get, and gets only what they pay for, where those who have money can have much but those who have had to struggle to have the little money they have must often go without. We strove to achieve a more social form of community than that.

In paying the fees the students contributed towards the financial needs of the college. It was intended that this, together with other income the college managed to generate, would be enough to cover the total running costs for the year. Within this the college provided everything that students needed to live and study for the three terms of the year. Only if students wanted to go beyond the basics that were provided, to buy such items as books for themselves rather than borrow from the library, to buy extra food or make personal telephone calls, did they have to pay individually. We tried to achieve quite practically something of the family situation where each child is given, within the means available to the particular family, what they individually need—because they are loved—and where the children also participate, according to their age and nature, in the work of the household. But of course we were not the parents, nor the students our children. A free relationship between students and staff had to be maintained. The students were mature adult people, sometimes older and with more experience in their particular fields than their teachers.

Tuition Fees

The name 'tuition fee' is not strictly correct but it was the name we used as having meaning for people not yet come to the recognition that education cannot have a cost in the way an economic product does. As I indicated more fully in the last chapter, what the student pays as tuition fee and the teacher receives as salary can only be truly understood when considered as gift or contribution rather than as sale and purchase. Education is not an economic product; to think in those terms is an economic unreality. To treat it as such distorts the true relationship between the teacher and the student. The student does not buy education. Just as the salary is a contribution to the teacher to enable him to live so that he can teach, so the fee is a contribution by the students to the running costs of the college so that they can study at the college. It is not a free gift but a 'contracted contribution'—the student contracts to contribute an agreed sum and the college contracts to run certain courses to which the student has the right to attend.

It is basically true to say that, in the main, the full cost of a course is incurred when the first student signs up. This total cost does not increase in any material way when others join. So it cannot truly be said that there is a cost for each student, or that if a student pays only half the fee then there is an unpaid balance that someone else must pay. In fact whatever a person contributes will help towards the whole and so reduce what others need to contribute. The idea or concept that the fee asked of the student is a contribution towards the total cost of running the course is much closer to the actual economic facts than to think of it as the cost of one more person in the course, which it is not.

If that is accepted, how does one arrive at a system where everyone makes a contribution rather than a payment or purchase? Should everyone make the same contribution, and if so why? People have often said that it is unfair if some people are accepted on a contribution lower than others in the same course; it means that those who pay more are subsidizing those who contribute less. But that would be true only if there was an actual cost which I have shown there is not. What do we mean by fair? Is it fairer that everyone pays the same mathematical amount irrespective of their life's circumstances, their social background, and their financial possibilities? Or is it fairer that a person be asked to make a contribution relative to his life's circumstances? Can one really assert that it is fair that a student, coming from a poor country where the standard fee would be equal to more than a year's earnings, pay the same as a student from an economically wealthy country where the fee can be earned in, say, one month? Emerson College set out to be a world college. Should not something of the diversity of the world situation be reflected in the fees charged to students from that world? We have to overcome the deeply ingrained thinking in our society according to which education is similar to an economic product that has a cost which has to be paid.

Students came from many and varied cultures and life situations and through quite different destinies. It added greatly to the life, experience, and culture of the college to have as widespread a cross-section of world humanity as possible, and if a person paid even a small amount, that small amount was a contribution to the whole and so reduced what was required from others. The ideal would be that students contributed according to their ability to pay, that is, according to their situation in life. But the great majority of prospective students, coming from the wider world as it is, would neither have the way of thinking nor the concepts to enable them to work with such ideas before they had actually been to the college, certainly not sufficiently to take them into their will forces. Students needed to know the cost of coming to the college before they committed themselves. They had to know how much to earn, or to ask for in a grant application. That is the way of the world. We had to specify the actual fee in the college prospectus. So, though we had to state a fee as the cost of coming to the college in a form that would be understood by the world at large, we did try to do it in a way that would give some suggestion of a different approach to such questions, and to say that if their will to come was serious but their financial resources limited they should let us know.

We were sometimes told that people do not learn the value of things if they do not have to pay directly for them. There is, of course some truth in this, but only in the short term. What they usually learn is not the true value of what they buy but its monetary value. This leads to a valuing of things that are directly paid for, but a carelessness and wasting of those things that are not so paid for. Learning to live by the true value of things rather than their nominal monetary value is an important moral step. For students intending to set out on a path of inner development every step along that path has to be accompanied by a development of moral understanding and inner discipline. Providing for students in the way we did within the particular social life of the college gave them the opportunity to learn to value what was given and free rather than only what was paid for.

Irrespective of the course attended there were two standard rates, a higher one for the first year and a lower one for the second and any subsequent years. In practice, particularly for their first year, we asked the students to pay the fee as published. Most students whose will to attend the college was strong, when pressed, were able to find more money than they first thought. Some might even be persuaded to first earn more money and come a year later. But there were always a few who without some reduction would not manage and for these we always considered a reduction of the fee.

What has just been said applied in its fullest sense only to the tuition element of the fee. But there were, except for a very few, the additional costs of room and meals. These were related to actual economic costs and so were more truly purchases. Whereas, if a student could not pay the tuition fee it would not actually cost the college more than a minimal amount to accept him, if he did not pay the board and lodging there would be actual costs. So, although we always tried to obtain the full tuition fee, if we felt that a potential student was strong in his intentions we might accept him and agree a lower tuition contribution. But we would normally try to get them to pay the actual costs of board and lodging.

There were times when we accepted students without any contribution towards fees at all: young people with special destinies who found their way to the college along difficult paths, people who Francis or others felt might be just those for whom the college was created. That they had not got the money could not be a reason to refuse them. Often through connections and friends of the college we found someone who would make a contribution, at least to cover board and lodging, but sometimes we merely absorbed any cost into the general college overheads. If we accepted it as true what Francis said of the college being willed by the spiritual world itself for the special young people of that time, then how could we refuse such a student just because he did not have the money. My experience was that Francis himself when not sure of a new applicant preferred to accept the wrong person into the college than refuse someone 'for whom the college was created'. Certainly we did not always get it right. But, as I indicated above, over most of the early years our income more than covered our costs which suggested that we could not have got it very wrong. In those days our most effective publicity was by word of mouth of the students themselves. Right up into the late 1980s there was very little actual publicity other than by Francis's and other teachers' lecture tours and the college prospectus. In fact, in our accounts we did not even have an account for publicity until 1987.

For the second and subsequent years it was possible to work more freely. By then we knew the students. Their values and perception of life had probably changed. I frequently had conversations with students who wanted to return to a training course but who did not have the financial means. I would often end by giving them a target figure which they would need somehow to earn, beg or borrow for us to accept them. How far this target was set above, or on rare occasions below, their original estimates of what they could come up with depended on my and the teachers' judgement of their intentions and their inner resolves. It was surprising how often they did manage to bridge the difference, or at least make a real attempt to do so. There were times when we would accept someone who had made determined efforts but where there was no certainty as to how much they would eventually achieve. Sometimes we did not actually know until the end of the year what they would finally be able to pay.

Behind all this was our intention that if a student came with serious questions, a true impulse and the will to work, then we would not let his financial situation, or the lack of any scholarship funds alone prevent his coming to the college.

Rents

The level of rents were set in the first place by what we had to pay landladies in the village to obtain the number of rooms we needed in order to survive. As our own student housing offered considerable benefits over the rooms in the village we felt, to be fair, we had to charge slightly more. I look at this in more detail in the next chapter.

Meals

The finances of providing meals was a little different. In this there was minimal capital outlay. The main costs were the running costs, salaries for the cooks, provisions, power, and the replacement of crockery, pots, pans, and ovens, etc. This facility was not just a means of providing meals for students. As I mentioned earlier, the meals, sitting down together, played a very important part in the social and educational life of the college for both students and staff. Staff were encouraged to at least join the community for lunch, the main meal of the day. For staff eating at the college with the students was part of the life and work of the college. Refreshments at mid-morning and afternoon breaks were not charged for but were free for everyone, including visitors and friends. There were also, usually, four festive meals during the year that were provided for everyone, including families and those who did not normally eat at the college.

So the costs of running the kitchen had two elements: meals for students which they paid for under 'board', and that which could be said to be a part of the life of the college as a whole and treated as part of the overheads. As I have shown, the tuition fee did not just relate to the tuition element but was aimed at covering the general cost of running the college. This second part then came under the general running costs and so properly could be included within the tuition fee.

Another factor was something I touched on in chapter 13. Sharing in the meals was not something separate from the educational experience of life at the college. Also, Francis had always said that healthy food was essential for the students if they were to benefit fully from what they learnt in the classroom. This led to the question: should part of the actual costs of providing meals for students be included in overheads so as to reduce the possible savings that would encourage students to opt out of having college meals? It would be better for the student and the college if, where a student could not afford the full fees including meals, the tuition element of the fee was reduced by the college rather than savings be made by the students not eating properly.

If a student opted out of some meals there was, in reality, only a small saving to the college, the overheads could not be reduced proportionately. In the same way, one extra person having meals was not a full increase in cost. There was a good case for putting part of the running costs of the kitchen into overheads, so reducing the charge for meals to nearer the actual cost of the food. This was something that a few of us would have liked to have done more extensively, but on the Council there was also a feeling for the conventional wisdom that actual costs should be paid for, not subsidized by the tuition fee, so what we could do was sometimes limited.

17
Developments and New Buildings

In this chapter I shall give a brief survey of the growth of Emerson up until the late 1980s, through the development of the outer physical body of the college. That is, through the building and acquisition of new property and of related developments. This gives a picture of remarkably strong growth during those years. Some of this will have been touched on earlier in the book but I repeat it here to give a complete picture.

The original purchase in 1967 consisted of Pixton House and campus including the stable-block, Old Orchard Cottage, and the Lodge on the Hartfield Road. A temporary wooden hut for large meetings and eurythmy was acquired that first summer. Though temporary it is still there and well used. Tablehurst Farm, taken over the following year, consisted of about 200 acres of farm land; some run-down farm buildings: and two cottages, one of which was reputed to be over 400 years old. There were a further two semi-detached farm cottages and a 30-acre piece of farmland—the Windmill Cottages and fields—on the north end of the farm which, at £20,000 on top of the basic cost, was felt to be too great a commitment. Manning Goodwin then stepped in and purchased this property in order to protect that high end of the farm. He gave the use of the land and houses to the college free of any charge. It was his hope that later the college would be in a position to buy them from him, which we were able to do in 1973.

Manning Goodwin played an important part in this development so I should say something here about him. Manning came from America. His mother, Anne Stockton, was a teacher in the New York Steiner School. When as a young man he was uncertain as to his next step in life Anne persuaded him to go to Emerson. In 1966, the last year in the Huts, he came with his young family to join the Foundation Year. Manning was deeply impressed by Francis and set out to support the college he had founded. He was of enormous help in dealing with the practical aspects of the developing college and played an important part in the acquisition of its new home in Pixton. He was asked to be one of the founding members of the reformed legal body of The Emerson College Trust Ltd in 1967. Manning had inherited a considerable amount of money, but used little of this for himself. He felt that he had been given it in trust to use for the community. I will speak more of his contributions later in this chapter.

After five years in often problematic rented accommodation, the college had taken the important step of buying its own property, Pixton, mainly in the form of land on which it could build. The existing buildings were quite inadequate for its purpose. So now came the need to plan for the future; to decide what buildings would be required. Francis invited Rex Raab, an architect and an anthroposophist whose architecture he greatly respected, to take on the design of the new building. One problem was that Rex, though English by birth, lived and worked in Germany so he could not be present at Emerson as often as would be necessary.

The original plan was that the college would move into Pixton during the summer of 1968, a year after the purchase. The main reason for this delay was the lack of facilities and space to provide meals for the 80 to 90 students and staff that could be expected. So the first building urgently needed was a kitchen and dining-room block. But before this could be planned some idea of how many it would eventually have to cater for and, more particularly, where it should be placed within the overall plan was needed. For that some sort of overall development plan would have to first be made. But to develop such a plan some idea of probable future growth was needed. All this would take more than one year, and at present there was, anyway, no money for it. A further question was that when money was available should it really be spent on some grand dining-room complex rather than on teaching spaces or a hall?

Supported by Anthony Kaye it was decided that the present kitchen in Pixton could be adapted to cooking for quite a large number (in later years over 220 were catered for in that kitchen) and the main rooms in Pixton could, for the present, serve two purposes, teaching and dining. That eased the time pressure and the college then could move straight away in 1967. But there was still the problem of the overall plan.

After the initial huge effort in the summer of 1967 to get the new campus far enough ready to move the college in and get it running, the next important step was a serious look at the future needs. Francis and Rex Raab invited Arne Klingborg to assist in this. Arne had founded Steinerhögskolan, a college similar in purpose to Emerson, in Järna, Sweden, also in 1962. He was a dynamic man, an artist and himself an architect, so his help was very much valued.

* * *

Francis saw the Foundation Year Course as preparation for the training courses which would lead into work in the world. His work had been in Waldorf education and perhaps influenced by this he saw a hall and stage for drama and eurythmy, and for meetings of the whole community, as of central importance. Rex out of his experience in designing schools also saw this, and he saw it in terms of a grand building that stood as a statement of its purpose. But before such a building could be thought of, the overall plan had to be worked out. This required an idea of what other buildings would be needed. Here was the problem.

In planning a school there is much that is calculable. The number and size of classrooms and the subjects to be covered can all be more or less known in advance. So an overall development plan can be worked out early in the process. To a certain extent the same is true for any particular training course. Francis and Rex wanted to do this for Emerson. But Emerson was not like a school. The Foundation Year was over half the college. It was impossible to see how that was going to unfold in the future. Every year the students were new and brought different questions and different impulses. And out of this what training courses would eventually develop?

In the early years several attempts were made to think through how Emerson would develop and to foresee future needs and so come to an overall plan for the campus. This always included a substantial hall with stage and auditorium for drama and eurythmy. But life showed that Emerson would not develop out of any predetermined plans but only out of the individual impulses and intuitions of the many people who came to carry the work, and through the many questions and differing needs of the students who came.

Emerson was an organization that by its nature was open to the future and to the people, both staff and students, and sometimes others, who were enabled to awaken their deeper impulses, often to bring these to fruition at the college. Who, at that time, could have known or even imagined how the college was going to unfold, what different courses or events would be started? And would a purpose-built hall and stage have served in the way that Ruskin, with all its inadequacies, has done? Looking back over all the events that have taken place in that hall from carnivals, festivals, dances, Christmas dinners for the whole community in one room, plays, eurythmy performances, House Meetings, concerts, and other such gatherings where we could sit facing either the stage, the window, the screen, or in a circle, one must ask how all these that were an essential part of the life of the college could have been achieved in a hall specially designed for drama and eurythmy. Ruskin Hall was the social centre where people met for all the events involving the whole community. Yet, as I shall explain later, it was really a hodgepodge originally designed as two art studios but adapted to a stage and auditorium. It seems to have been part of the destiny of the college to have, over the years, many different architects who have tried to bring design and form into the campus, but somehow events have always overtaken them.

As Rex Raab lived and worked in Germany it was envisaged that a local architect was needed to do the detail and supervision of the necessary alterations to existing buildings and later the on-site work of new construction. Lambert Gibbs, who lived in Forest Row, agreed to do this. But Lambert was an award-winning architect in his own right, so had ideas of his own. He had no connection to anthroposophy itself, but was interested in the sort of architecture that it inspired. So in reality Lambert became the main architect with Rex more in the role of consultant. Lambert dealt with the many alterations to Pixton House and grounds as well as the drive and new car park that were put in place during that first summer. Another man very involved in the building developments over the years was Colin Packington as the quantity surveyor. Colin had been a pupil of Michael Hall School and Francis Edmunds had been his class-teacher, so he had a particular interest in the college and was a real help over the following years.

But before the new main building could be started, the car park and Karnant were completed.

Car Park

In planning the campus it was decided to keep cars, particularly car parking, to the periphery on the north side. As this was a site on the hill which could then be seen from some miles down the Medway Valley to the east the planning authorities insisted it was sunken and surrounded by trees.

Karnant

After the move to Pixton the first new building to go up was a house for the Edmunds. For the first 18 months they lived in Pixton House in the rooms that later became the library. The new house was funded by the sale of Kinnerton where they had lived during the time in the Huts. Karnant, as they named the new house, was designed by Rex Raab.

Ruskin, Birch and Maple

After much discussion it was eventually planned to start the main building programme with one classroom block and two separate student houses—each with eight single rooms. The classroom block would include two large rooms with north-facing high windows for the arts and eurythmy. Below these would be a number of study and craft rooms and some sort of science laboratory facilities. The building, later named Ruskin, was designed to be erected at minimum cost but providing maximum basic usable space.

The cost was originally estimated at about £72,000. This was a very large sum of money, more than Pixton and Tablehurst Farm combined had cost. A considerable number of gifts and friendly loans had been received from supporters, particularly in America. But by January 1969 it had become clear that in order to go ahead £45,000 still needed to be found. It was agreed that the college would extend its bank borrowing. A clause would be included in the building contract to enable us to stop the work before completion if necessary. The basic design of Ruskin was created by Rex Raab, but the details and the design of the student houses were the work of Lambert Gibbs.

I remember how, at the Council Meeting on 1 January 1969, after much discussion, Francis asked each member present in turn whether we should go ahead, that is, to take on a loan of £45,000 to complete the buildings. Each member spoke and each agreed that we should do so. The building contract was put out to tender and the contract offered to Ringmer Building Works Ltd. The tender, though the cheapest, was higher than expected. Some items had to be omitted to reduce cost. The contract was signed in early March and actual building work started a week or so later. The two student houses, later named Birch and Maple, were completed in good time and occupied during the autumn term of 1969. But the classroom block, Ruskin, which should have been completed by the end of that year, was considerably delayed by continual problems. It did not help that the builder's site-foreman had a drink problem. At one point work almost ground to a halt due to poor organization leading to lack of materials. Things went better when the foreman was eventually replaced by the promotion of one of the joiners on the project. There was a major fault in the insulation sheaths of the underground heating pipes which then all had to be dug up and replaced, and I never quite understood how the building came to be about a foot lower than planned! This meant that the paving around it was the same level as the road. An embarrassment to those involved, but actually having certain advantages to the college.

With the new foreman the situation and the whole mood on the site greatly improved. I got to know many of the workmen quite well. Towards the end, during the summer term of 1970, when preparations for Shakespeare's *The Tempest* were being rehearsed in the unfinished new hall with workmen still active in the room, one of them told me that they were going on a 'go slow'. When I looked worried and appalled he said, 'We like it here, we don't want to leave.'

Finally the building was completed at the end of June 1970 in time for the end-of-term public performances of *The Tempest*, a great success and the first of many Shakespeare plays. The room intended for laboratory facilities became the Agriculture Course and research space. The two art rooms were transformed so as to be usable as a temporary raised stage and auditorium as well as a general meeting and multi-purpose space. This temporary arrangement actually became permanent. They were extremely useful and adaptable spaces and over the years provided room for many and varied functions—even a Mayfair on one really wet occasion! It also became the home of the Foundation Year whose numbers were later often well into the 90s.

We now had 16 new student rooms on campus and a very considerable extension of the classroom spaces. This made an enormous change to the life of the college which had become extremely cramped. During 1969–70 there had been 87 students. This increased to some 130 for the year 1970–71, so actually there continued to be a shortage of spaces.

Doc's Dip—connecting Pixton to the Farm

When Pixton and Tablehurst Farm were purchased there was no direct easy connection between them apart from a rough footpath across the stream that divided the two. Vehicle access was a long way round through the village, a distance of nearly two miles. The Waters family had originally lived in Tablehurst Manor on the village side of the farm. Keeping the farm they later sold the Manor and bought Pixton House and fields, but never established a vehicular connection to the farm. Jimmy Waters told me that he had tried to dam the stream but heavy rains had always washed the dam away. Now, the earth from the car park excavation, and later that from the cutting into the bank for Ruskin, was used to construct a causeway across the stream to the farm.

To jump ahead a few years to complete the story of this causeway, the culvert of three concrete sections placed under it for the stream to run through was not secured properly and soon began to shift as the water dug round it. We had a student at that time, John Docherty, an older and very unusual man. He had a deep connection with nature, or should I say, with the elemental beings in nature. He was widely read and a man of very great wisdom on many subjects. When the causeway threatened to give way he hired a digger and for several days he dug out the clay in and around the stream, sealed up the culvert and strengthened the whole embankment so turning the causeway into a dam. The lake so created was often referred to as 'Doc's Dip', or sometimes 'Loch Docherty'. The lake has never shown any sign of erosion. John succeeded where both Jimmy Waters and the builders failed.

Plaw Hatch and Busses Farms

In 1970 there were two developments in the area which though not of Emerson College itself did arise out of it in that they were purchases by former Emerson students still connected in different ways to the college. One was the purchase of Plaw Hatch Farm by Manning Goodwin. Plaw Hatch was a dairy farm of some 143 acres with fairly old buildings. Manning set about converting it into a biodynamic dairy farm. He intended that it would work closely with the Agriculture Course at Emerson and with Tablehurst Farm. Manning himself had little previous farming experience. This farm comes back into the story later.

The other development started when Jimmy and Pauline Anderson, a couple who had just completed the Agriculture Course, purchased Busses Farm, near East Grinstead. They were both very socially-minded people who had already farmed in Scotland. They saw a farm as very much a community affair and Busses became not only an active farm but also a centre of social activities. Unfortunately, due to the particular legal arrangements that had been entered into in setting up the farm, some years later it was not possible to continue and it had to be sold and the Andersons moved back to Scotland.

The Architects Partnership

In 1971 the college began looking for another local architect. John Davy had become involved in the college development by now and with him it was felt we needed someone local who worked more actively out of anthroposophy than Lambert Gibbs was able to. Christian Thal-Jantzen was a young recently-qualified architect who though already involved in architecture had not yet established himself in a practice. He was actively involved in anthroposophy and was committed to bringing the Spirit to expression in his design work. He had interesting ideas and also connections with other young architects. He had recently established a connection with another young architect named Tom Rowling.

After discussions with him and Rex Raab it was agreed that Christian would become a part-time member of the staff of the college, initially for one year. He would work an average of two-and-a-half days a week for the college which would provide him with a room he could use as an office. Rex Raab would act as a 'tutor consultant' and would work with Christian so that the college would still, in an overall way, benefit from Rex's great experience and knowledge. Over the next few years Christian invited a number of other young architects to join him. As well as Tom Rowling these included at different times Jørgen Mosbaek, Bill Chase, Wolodymyr Radysh, and Tony Cooper—then director of the first year at the Canterbury School of Art and Architecture.

The planning authorities had indicated that they would not agree any new buildings until there was an acceptable outline overall plan for the campus. This was to be the new architects' first task and it again led to many discussions as to the future shape and size of the college. All that could be imagined at that time was a college of between 200 to 300 students, of whom probably at least half would be in the Foundation Year.

In addition they took on a number of alterations to existing buildings such as the extension to the old stable-block.

Ruskin Extension and Pixton Builders

It had always been planned to extend Ruskin. The need for the additional space this would provide was urgent. We now had our own architects' group. In 1973 the idea was put forward of also initiating a building group. Apart from the possibility of this being cheaper, what was of particular interest was that it might be set up in a way that enabled some students to earn their fees working on the site. One of the architects, Tom Rowling, who also had an interest in the building activity itself, expressed interest and offered to start the group. Don Ratcliffe and Jonathan Soper, both former students and practical young men joined him. So the Pixton Builders was founded. They were set up as an independent business, not part of the college, but arising out of it. They did a number of alterations and minor constructions round the campus, including what later became the first-floor sculpture studio in the stable-block, before tackling the Ruskin extension.

The Ruskin extension included two classroom spaces—a weavery and the Education Course room—as well as two study rooms or course offices, and a small art or craft room. It would also house a boot room and the new boilers in the cellar. Planning permission was obtained and work by Pixton Builders started in the autumn of 1973. After some student involvement, a few ups and downs and delays, the building was completed and opened on Saturday 23 September 1975, the 13th birthday of the college.

In 1977 when there were no plans for new building in the near future the Architects Partnership and Pixton Builders both moved out of the Emerson Campus into William Morris Yard in the village, a property Manning Goodwin had purchased and now made available to them. In 1982 the Architects Partnership was dissolved. David Austin, who had more recently joined the partnership, continued to do work for the college.

Christian Thal-Jantzen, Christopher Budd, and Manning Goodwin had founded the Hoathly Hill Community in 1972. They now became more fully involved in developing this. From his experience at Emerson College Christian had became particularly interested in working with money, capital, and land in the light of anthroposophy. Christian also had in mind something Francis Edmunds used to speak of as being needed for difficult times that lay ahead for human society—that is, what he called 'Oasis of Cultural'. He and Christopher also founded an organization, 'Land and Capital Exchange'.

Colour for Building

This was founded, also in William Morris Yard, by Robert Lord, a former student, Peter Horsfall, and Francis Gregory.

Tablehurst New Barn

In 1972, with the aid of a government grant a large barn was built on the farm. This was used mainly for winter housing of the animals and for hay-drying and storage in summer and autumn.

106 Hartfield Road

When Herbert and Ursula had joined the college the house at 106 Hartfield Road had been rented for them. This house was put up for sale by the owners in 1973 and the college purchased it for £11,000 to enable the Koepfs to continue living there. We had to take out a bank mortgage to help finance this. The saving in rent covered bank interest.

Windmill Cottages and Fields

Juan Berlin, who lived in Mexico, was an old friend and supporter of Francis Edmunds. He financed a number of young people from Mexico to attend the college. In 1973 he lent the college money to enable it to purchase from Manning the two semi-detached houses and the 30 acres of land at the top end of the farm. As I mentioned earlier, Manning had purchased these in order to save them for the college when it could afford them. He now sold them to the college for £20,000, the original cost to him. Although the college and farm had had the free use of them before this they were now secured for the future.

The Cyrnel Bakery

The year 1974 saw much activity towards setting up the Cyrnel Bakery. For some years the college had been baking its own bread, the wheat now coming from our own farm. Many friends in the neighbourhood frequently expressed a desire to buy this bread. In the autumn of 1972 a young American, Robert Koerber, had come to study in the Foundation Year. He was a skilled baker having served an apprenticeship under a German master-baker before working for an established bakery in the USA. But he had decided to stop baking and take up painting. Sometime earlier Manning Goodwin had purchased a building in the village which had been a repair shop. He had recognized its potential but had not yet found a purpose for it. Now there was a need for bread, a supply of biodynamic wheat from Tablehurst and Busses Farms, a potential baker, and possible premises. What we needed was to find some capital to bring it all about and to persuade Robert, who was presently attending the Painting Course, to take up baking again. Through a public meeting and an appeal we managed to raise enough donations and loans. Robert agreed to commit himself to the enterprise for three years. He actually stayed for nearly five. The bakery opened in early 1975.

Robert had studied Steiner's lectures *World Economy* and the threefold social order with me and was interested in, so far as possible, setting up the bakery on these lines. The ownership of the land and buildings and the operation of baking were separated. The intention originally was to put the ownership of the land and buildings into a separate Trust. But for a number of reasons this was not possible at the time and so it was eventually decided that the college itself, having committed itself to the bulk of the loans, would own it 'in trust for the community'. The rent paid by the business would cover interest. In the event this was considerably more than covered. There were two important clauses in the lease. Firstly, the premises were rented to Robert Koerber personally, not to his company, and the arrangement could not be sold on by him to anyone else. Secondly, the premises were rented for the purpose of baking bread and other pastries 'using biodynamic flour so long as available and viable'. For the actual baking a separate independent limited company was formed: the Cyrnel Bakery of which Robert and his wife Janet were the two directors and sole shareholders. Robert put many hours of hard work into the baking and his bakery was much valued in the village. He told me once that he liked nothing better than to have a little old lady happily going out of his shop hugging a still warm loaf of healthy fresh bread. When Robert eventually left in 1979 the premises were rented to Rosa Gilder and Steve Moran under the same terms and so continued as originally intended.

A House for the Wilkes Family

Since they had arrived in 1968 the Wilkes family had lived in the attic of Pixton house. They now had two small children and it was urgent that they had a larger home. So after discussion it was decided to build a house for them on the campus. With some gifts for the purpose and loans it was now possible to do this. John Wilkes himself was able to also put money in for a flat for his mother.

The Yager Project

At the same time a friend in America, Gilbert Yager, had made a donation for a two-roomed flat for guest lecturers. His two daughters had been students of the college in 1963. Later he and his wife, Marie, visited in the Huts. They had also been the first to make a substantial gift towards the purchase of Pixton. Several further gifts were made during the following years. Marie had recently died leaving in her will $10,000 to the college. At the same time the Koepfs, still living in 106 Hartfield Road, wished to move on campus. It was decided to sell this house and put the money into the Yager Project for a staff flat for them. Molly von Heider had joined the college in 1973 and needed somewhere more permanent to live. She offered to sell her house in

Stourbridge and lend the money to the college to enable a three-bedroom flat to be included for herself.

So the Yager Project was got underway. The Wilkes house and small annexe was built as one unit and Molly von Heider's, the Koepf's, and the visiting lecturer's flat were built as another two-storey block. These were designed by the Architects Partnership and built by Pixton Builders. In order to obtain planning permission the college had to sign an undertaking that the accommodation would be used only as staff or student housing and designed in such a way that it could not be sold off as separate flats. Building work started in September 1975; it was completed in 1977, the main block earlier in the year, and later the Wilkes house. The final cost came to rather more than originally estimated. During 1975 the house at 106 Hartfield Road had been sold as planned, at a useful profit.

Old Plaw Hatch House

The Social Development Centre had been founded in 1975 and for the first year was run in a large private house lent by Manning Goodwin. In 1976 Old Plaw Hatch House came on the market and it was decided to buy this as the permanent home of the Centre. The agreed price was £50,000 of which £15,000 had already been found. The bank agreed an overdraft facility for the remaining £35,000 secured by a mortgage on the property. There was good prospect of finding more donations in the near future to reduce this borrowing. So the property was purchased and the Centre was able to move into its new home for its second year 1976–7.

The Eurythmy House

Francis and, more particularly, Elizabeth Edmunds were keen to have a purpose-built eurythmy room. A large sum of money for this purpose had been raised by them from friends in America, Switzerland, Germany, and England. The architect David Austin designed the building. This was done within the overall plan which included a theatre. The eurythmy building would be part of the theatre complex. Building by Pixton Builders started in July 1977 and was completed within the year.

Plaw Hatch Farm

As I mentioned above, Plaw Hatch Farm had been bought by Manning Goodwin who developed it as a biodynamic dairy farm with a milk-round of unpasteurised organic milk. He had hoped to work in connection with the agriculture programme at Emerson, as well as having apprentices on the farm. But this had not worked well and difficulties had arisen. He was very much involved elsewhere and could not give it the attention needed. So he eventually decided to pull out and sell the farm, hopefully to a buyer who could continue developing what he had started. After much discussion and even public meetings it became clear that there was then no person or organization able to take over the farm in order to save it from being sold on the open market. This would mean losing the milk-round of healthy untreated milk, the supply of biodynamic vegetables to the Seasons shop as well as all that had been achieved in turning it into a biodynamic farm.

Within the Council of Management the need to save the farm was also felt strongly. But there was concern that it was not within the proper task of the college to run two farms, nor did we have the people that could manage it. Those running Tablehurst were all fully involved there and they themselves did not have the experience also to take on a very different kind of farm. Another important consideration was that the college did not have the capital to buy the farm. But Manning was prepared to wait for the money. He made a very generous offer which the college finally accepted. This was that the college would purchase the land consisting of 105 acres of dairy farmland and woodland, farm buildings, the annexe, bothy and stable-block, and the live and dead-stock for a total of about £125,000. The college would pay approximately £4,000 per annum for 20 years and would make a final payment of approximately £90,000 in 20 years' time. The £90,000 being the balance of £45,000 plus a maximum of another £45,000 to cover interest and depreciation in money value.

The college took over the running of the farm on 1 April 1977. Chuck Beedy and David Adams, and later Craig Cook, were eventually taken on to run it. Both Chuck and Craig were former students of the college. They were all keen young men but without extensive farm management experience. Towards the end of two years it became clear that the farm was not working well and could not be made viable without considerably more capital which the college did not have. There were also social problems within the farm. Early in 1979 Christian Thal-Jantzen and Christopher Budd, two trustees of the Hoathly Hill Community, offered to take over the arrangement with Manning Goodwin. After discussions with them and with Manning it was agreed that the college would give up the farm. Manning came to a new arrangement with Christian and Christopher to take over the farm from 1 April 1979. They ran the farm for a year, but it became apparent that they would not find the necessary capital to enable Manning to pull out. Bob Wills and others of St Anthony's Trust were then able to raise sufficient capital from the anthroposophical bank in Bochum, Germany, for St Anthony's Trust to take over the farm land and buildings and to also run the farm activity.

The college could feel satisfied with the outcome. The farm had been saved and was now in the hands of others who would continue to develop it as originally intended. The venture had cost the college between £1,000 and £2,000, a cheap price to pay for what was achieved.

Parklands Fields

At this time the college was also able to take over the Parkland fields, that is, the fields to the west and south of Pixton House as far as the river. These had been tenanted by a farmer, Mr Johnson, prior to purchase by the college, but it was only now possible to obtain the use of them.

Student Housing

By this time student numbers at Pixton had risen to over 180 and looked to increase further. Housing them was a very real problem. There were still only the 16 purpose-built rooms on campus and some rooms in Shalesbrooke. It depended very heavily on finding rooms with landladies in the village. In 1974 this difficult and important work had been passed over from Roswitha Spence to Myra and Alistair Macdonald and, later, also Rachel Horsfall. Consideration was given to the possibility of building a block with between 60 and 100 student rooms, but the cost was far too high to contemplate at present. It would be cheaper to buy houses in the village, though more expensive to run. There were also more student families needing accommodation. Through the generosity of a Canadian student, Jadie Hassell, who on returning home after completing her course offered to sell us her house in Forest Row on very generous terms, and with financial help from many others, we were able to purchase Silver Ridge in September 1978. This then housed another Canadian family and three students for the year 1978–9.

Then during 1979, with further financial support and bank loans, we purchased three more houses: 119 Hartfield Road, 13 Post Horn Lane, and 16 Highfields. The latter was also from a former student returning home and offered on generous terms. Martlet, a large house on the Lewes Road, was also offered at a very low rent by a friend. Martlet was able to house around six students.

Tablehurst Barn Fire

In the late autumn of 1979 the new barn on Tablehurst Farm, full of the year's harvest of hay and straw, burnt down. The insurance treated it as a total loss although one end was included in a later building. With the insurance money and some gifts we put up a better and larger barn the following year.

Old Plaw Hatch Extension

In 1978 the student numbers in the Social Development Centre had reached 30 with signs that numbers might still grow. Old Plaw Hatch House did not provide all the spaces needed for their growing work, particularly for such activities as lectures and eurythmy. Following an appeal an extension was added to the house in 1979. This made an enormous difference and was a very welcome improvement to the life and work of the Centre.

More Houses

Two more houses were purchased in 1982. A house at 108 Hartfield Road was offered on favourable terms by a friend who was leaving the area, and 20 Freshfield Bank was purchased for Olive Whicher. Of the £39,500 price, £29,000 was an interest-free loan available so long as Olive continued to live there. This amount was eventually made into a gift. In 1982, when Ilse Brice, the Housemother retired Molly von Heider suggested that her third bedroom and utility room in the Yager building be converted into a flat for Ilse. Ann Gooding who had been working in the office for many years lent £12,000 at minimal interest towards the cost of the conversion. In March 1983, 8 Post Horn Lane was purchased for £33,000 and in 1988, 9 Post Horn Lane was purchased.

Westwood and Oaktree

At the end of 1981 we began to plan for building a student block of 24 single student rooms and a staff flat. We decided at this time that all future large buildings, especially students blocks, should include at least one staff flat. We had just recently received a substantial legacy from Lionel Elin. With loans from Mercury Provident Pension Fund, the Anthroposophical Society, bank borrowing, and an appeal, we were confident we could cover the estimated £220,000 cost. David Austin was commissioned to design it. We also decided for this building to go to conventional builders.

Tenders for the building were invited. The cheapest was fairly well above the estimates, but with some changes to the plans and simplification of the requirements we eventually got the price down to a reasonable figure, though still above the original estimates. Building started at the end of 1982. This was one building operation that went smoothly and without serious delay or problem. The site-foreman, Mr Derek Braidon, was a remarkably capable person. The building was completed and handed over on 19 December 1984.

In 1990 Oaktree, with 12 student's rooms and two staff flats, was completed. At this point, in addition to Pixton House, Ruskin, the Eurythmy House, and the converted stable-block there were on the campus itself four student housing blocks accommodating 52 students plus 11 staff houses or flats. In addition there were the two Windmill cottages and two farm houses on Tablehurst. The college had also purchased eight houses in the village. This came to a total of 23 houses or flats and 52 student rooms.

Paying for these Developments

I should say something about the financing of these developments, particularly of the student and staff housing.

Over the years many donations and legacies were received, some quite large, a few of which I have already described. Here again I would mention Charlotte Parker, of Spring Valley, because without her support for Francis it is hard to imagine how much could have been achieved. Nancy Laughlin was another American friend who gave very substantially. But there were very many smaller and different forms of giving which contributed very substantially to this growth.

The support for this new impulse of Francis Edmunds's was extraordinarily deep and widespread. Many people wanted to connect themselves with it in order to support the work with the young people who came. I have already said something of the many summer volunteer workers who came over the years and contributed with their work and the visiting teachers who gave a substantial part of what the students valued so much but who asked for little or no money in return. From early on I had a sense that the good times would not last and we had to put all our resources into property while we could, and to do this in a way that would be a source of income in the later difficult times that would surely come. We were then still in the pioneer stage—life would inevitably get more expensive. Also we could not expect that new people joining the staff in future times would be prepared to work so long and hard and for as little salary as those in the earlier phase.

The rents from our student rooms helped to pay the cost of their acquisition. We had to offer a reasonably high rent to landladies in the village in order to find enough rooms for all students who needed one. Landladies did not provide meals or cooking facilities, these were available in the college. But students in college houses, whether on campus or in houses owned or rented in the village, had the advantage that they could cook for themselves. We could not charge less for our own rooms than what students had to pay landladies in the village. In fact we charged slightly more to balance the benefits.

Each year I calculated the actual cost of heat and light; supply and laundering of sheets etc.; repairs and maintenance; and a share of management, and house-care costs. The rent paid above this was transferred each year into the housing fund to go towards paying off costs of building or buying accommodation. With 16 rooms on campus and up to 25 in the village this added up to a considerable sum. When later we began to build more student rooms on campus the capital costs not covered by gifts were all covered in this way. In the same way, a nominal rent from staff housing, after deducting actual costs, was put into the housing fund.

In the year 1989–90, after deducting all actual running costs, the surplus of rent income for the year that could be transferred to the housing fund for paying off the capital costs of building was £29,040. To give an idea of money value at that time, two years earlier 9 Post Horn Lane had been purchased for £44,000.

In 1987–8, after deducting the rent surplus the college made its first deficit on the income and expenditure account since 1969–70. In the future the surplus on the rent income would have increasingly to be used to cover running costs rather than development.

18
Tablehurst Farm

I have already given some details of the purchase and takeover of Tablehurst Farm but I think a fuller picture still needs to be given. In many ways the story of the farm could be a book in itself, but here I will give only a very brief idea of its start and early days.

Katherine Castelliz and Jeremy Kent were the two people whom Francis had invited to get the farm started. Katherine was an older woman deeply committed to anthroposophy and biodynamic agriculture, and with many years' experience, mainly with animals. Jeremy was a young man very committed to the care of the environment. As already described, though Pixton and Tablehurst Farm were purchased in summer 1967, the farm was not actually taken over until March 1968. Katherine moved into the small old 16th century cottage in the centre of the farm, but Jeremy preferred to continue living in one of the attic rooms in Pixton. There was another more modern cottage close to the village but this did not become available for some months and then was used to house a student family, Peter and Marsalaidh Clark. The farm was then very much part of the college and many students enjoyed some involvement in farm activities.

It was generally agreed that the purchase price of the farm had been low, but the condition of the buildings was poor and the soil fertility also very low. For five or six years the land had been repeatedly producing barley. Under the contract for purchase the vendor sowed the farm to grass before handing over. Only 65 per cent of this took and the rest had to be replanted. Katherine and Jeremy worked well together and built up a close working connection. Katherine was the older and had considerably more experience of biodynamic agriculture. She took overall responsibility for the animals while Jeremy for the arable work. There was very much work to be done in order to bring the land into health and the buildings and equipment into working order.

There was very little money available for purchase of equipment or livestock beyond an absolute minimum. Nine calves and an old and very second-hand tractor had already been acquired, but that was all they had to start with. More young animals were purchased at auction. This was a temporary measure to have some animals to fatten and to sell later. A regular herd would be founded once the farm was more established. It was later decided to build up a biodynamic herd of the beautiful red Sussex beef-cattle. In the meantime Jeremy hunted around for cheap second-hand equipment.

It was intended that the farm would be a mixed balance between a beef-herd, a small dairy herd to supply milk to the college, chickens, and part arable producing grain, vegetables, and sufficient hay for the animals. This would be supplemented by purchasing straw from the farm next door for winter bedding of the animals and the resulting manure.

In December 1968, nine months after taking over the farm, Francis was able to write in a progress report to all former Emersonians:

> *Down at the Farm, things are going forward also. Emerson now owns over 50 head of cattle (mostly young), the 5 young pigs are preparing to litter, the 80 laying hens are as industrious as ever, and the many pullets are eager to emulate their example as soon as nature makes them ripe for it. The first acres are under the plough, so that in the coming year we expect to have our own bio-dynamic supply of wheat for home-milling and bread-making. Meanwhile, the vegetable beds are well in hand, despite the marauding rabbits and invasions from the air. John Bradley, another returned Emersonian (he was with us the first term in Forest Row until his marriage) is now in charge of general maintenance. With the help of students, he has completed a very fine workshop down at the Farm, with a forge and other essential equipment, and room left over for setting up student metalwork again, we hope under Uwe Jacquet.*

The summer of 1968 was very wet. We did not have the necessary equipment for drying hay but with the use of tripods and Swedish fences and a considerable amount of labour supplied by our volunteer holiday workers, the yield of hay was an exceptionally fine one, both in quantity, some 80 tons, and above all in quality.

By autumn 1969 there were some 80 head of cattle for fattening and resale. As nucleus of a beef-herd several heifers had been acquired and there was the start of a milking-herd of Jersey cows; but as yet no proper milking equipment or building. The few cows ready were milked by hand by Katherine and her student assistants. The number of chickens had risen to 350—there was a ready market for the eggs in the village. The two acres of vegetables of 1968 were increased in 1969 to five acres. So, after one year, the farm was already supplying the college with some milk, vegetables, eggs, chicken, and beef.

Walter Rudert joined the staff in April 1969. He had been working on the biodynamic farm at Peredur and brought with him valuable experience. He moved with his wife Elli and young daughter Christiana into the second farm cottage. Elli, a lady of considerable wisdom, was an important addition to the farm. She also developed a very productive vegetable garden round their house. As already mentioned, Herbert Koepf joined the college in April 1970 and in September 1971 the full-time biodynamic Agriculture Course was founded. These events initiated gradual changes to the relationship of the farm to the college as well as to its direction and management. The students became involved and the farm staff played their parts in instructing them. There was also a gradual change in bringing the farm out of its pioneer stage and onto a more 'biodynamical professional' level. Though there was some improvement to the buildings and an acquisition of new machinery, this was still limited due to shortage of money.

In 1970 the purchase of Plaw Hatch Farm by Manning Goodwin and of Busses Farm by Jimmy and Pauline Anderson, all former students of the college, brought a wider co-operation between the various people involved. I have written more about them in chapter 17. To Katherine's disappointment, Plaw Hatch was set to become a biodynamic dairy farm with a milk-round of untreated milk. Tablehurst would now aim to be a mixed farm based on a beef-herd.

At the college itself there was a consciousness of, and interest in, these developments amongst both students and staff. They were of course periodically reported on and discussed at college meetings. The agricultural students found work experience on all the farms, and the Andersons, being very socially-minded people from Scotland, often organized community-orientated events and ceilidhs on their farm. On Tablehurst there were the occasional workdays for the whole college to help, for example, to harvest the potatoes and carrots. These occasions were an important coming together of the college and farm, and also an occasion when students worked beside teachers and farmers on a quite different level. During this time the farm took on two or three apprentices. They, as well as Jeremy, were still based at the college for their board and lodging, and the staff continued to join in much of the social life of the college.

In 1975 Robert Koerber at the Cyrnel Bakery started baking. Part of the impulse for this was to create a market for biodynamic flour. This called for an increase in grain production. At the beginning the mill for grinding the flour was set up on Busses, but when later that farm was sold the milling operation was moved to Tablehurst.

In the Progress Report of June 1976 John Davy wrote:

> *On a Saturday afternoon in the Summer Term, the staff gathers at Pixton for the annual farm walk. The sun usually shines, and we are fortified by hope of tea in Elli Rudert's garden at the end of the afternoon. After seven years I now count as a veteran farm-walker, and can make comparisons. This year the sun shone better than ever, and Southern England was parching in the most severe drought for 300 years. The fields still looked green, but there were deep cracks in the earth, and the grasses were beginning to flower and seed in early June, But despite these—for England—extreme conditions, the Tablehurst fields are in good heart. There is a quite unmistakable sense of life and strength returning to abused earth and of an organism regaining health. The higher pastures towards Windmill Cottage, which looked sad and poor a few years ago are now showing much richer growth. Our beautiful herd of dark chestnut Sussex cattle are beginning to outnumber the miscellaneous collections of animals with which the farm began. They fit the landscape wonderfully and thrive in our conditions.*
>
> *Parts of Minepits Wood have been cleared out, and Michael Spence has two hives of bees there. They have been a brief buzz away from a huge field of beans which seem to be ignoring the drought altogether and were thick with flower. So in mid June, while the Emerson College bee crew was still around, 80 pounds of honey were taken from these hives alone. It has a faint bean tang in the background, but is nevertheless delicious.*
>
> *As we walked, we found symptoms of the intensive work which our farm managers have put in, not only for the soil and animals, but for the details like fences, gates and water supplies. The whole farm is being worked through by human beings who love it, and the response is unmistakable. But we still have many old and patched-up buildings which we should dearly love to renew. The quality of the crops and livestock are beginning to show up the buildings. We hope we can find ways to make some real progress here before too long.*
>
> *Elli and Walter Rudert's cottage garden has also flourished and matured over the years, from being almost part of a rather exposed field, to become a sheltered composition of shrubs, roses, herbs and flowers. In this idyllic setting we got our tea—superb as always—and could give thanks for the blessing the farm brings for the College, and the new life which is coming into it.*

In 1977 both Katherine Castelliz and Jeremy Kent decided to leave. Jeremy wanted his own smallholding where he could work in his own way with nature on a smaller piece of land with minimal machinery. He was not really comfortable with the way the farm was developing under the influence of Emerson. Katherine was now in her 70s and wanted to be part of a smaller community which she joined in Wales with her old friends Marion Swatton, Mary Haydon, and Barbara Saunders Davies. Their going, in a certain way, brought to a final close the early pioneer days of the farm.

Hans-Peter Mader was invited to join the farm staff in December 1977. So the staff now consisted of Walther Rudert, Hans-Peter, and the apprentices, with Herbert Koepf as an adviser and guide. I was also involved in that the farm and college were closely linked financially. The main accounts were all maintained at the college, though Walther kept his own farm records. Though the accounts showed that the farm accumulated a profit over the years, this as well as further capital provided by the college was absorbed by the increase in the value of the growing livestock and the build-up of machinery. If all the livestock and machinery were sold then the college would recoup all that it had put in, but then it would have no productive farm.

* * *

Over the years the college and farm slowly developed their own identities. As the training courses grew in proportion to the whole, except for the Agriculture Course, there was a declining involvement of students in the farm and the connection became less and less important to the work of the college itself. While the importance of the farm produce for the college continued, its particular importance as the sole available source of biodynamic produce declined as it became increasingly possible to buy biodynamic or organic produce elsewhere. Its size also meant that it had to work on a larger scale than was needed by the college in order to be economically viable.

Francis had never really planned to acquire such a large farm. His idea was for land sufficiently large to provide for the needs of the Agriculture Course, to produce enough healthy food for the students and a place where Foundation Year students could experience working with nature. Over the years some of these needs came increasingly to be met by Annemarie's vegetable gardens on the college campus in a way that the farm could not match. By the mid-1980s the farm and college were really separate organisms with a relationship more like that of customer and supplier. Many of the staff had little or no direct relationship to the farm. Only the Agriculture Course continued a close working relationship.

Later, in the early '90s, the farm was properly separated off from the college and under the guidance of Peter Brown took on a new and vigorous life of its own. Its place within the local community and in the biodynamic movement was greatly strengthened.

But for Tablehurst Farm to develop into what it eventually became, Francis Edmunds had, as a matter of destiny rather than choice, to buy it together with Pixton, and for the college to start the process of transforming it into a working biodynamic farm. So another enterprise, founded and nurtured within Emerson College, grew up and achieved its free independent existence.

19
Summer Work, Workshops, and Short Courses

During the first few summers that followed the move to Pixton something of the life and mood of that first work-camp, which played such an important part in helping to get the house and campus ready, lived on. Without our having to advertise, the stream of young people wanting to join the work group continued. They came mostly from Europe but also from further afield, mainly young people in their early 20s. We always replied to their applications in the form that we understood they wished to come in order to help the college with their work. We provided board and lodging to make this possible, but no pay. The understanding was that they did not work to earn their board and lodging, but that this was provided to enable them to voluntarily work for the college. It was important to establish from the beginning that their help was a free deed. The work was full-time and as required and was often on the farm but also in the house, cleaning, painting and decorating, or in the garden.

In the earlier years there were no courses during the summers; everyone on campus was here working for the college—no one was here for themselves as they were, of necessity, during term time. Some past or continuing students stayed on and other prospective ones came, but they could only stay during the summer as fully committed workers, not as paying guests. In this way a very real feeling of community came about. It established an annual rhythmic balance between students being here in term time for, in the first place, their own inner needs, and the voluntary workers coming during the summer and working out of the needs of the college. These summer work-camps were, indeed, of very great benefit to the college, not just because so much necessary work was done but because it was given as a free deed. Something of this then lived on through the year in the spiritual environment of the college for the new students to come into. It was for the college a form of breathing in and breathing out.

The summers following the purchase of the farm were a time when Katherine Castelliz and Jeremy Kent were just getting started but without the necessary capital to buy anything beyond very basic machinery. Without this help much of the hay harvest of the first two summers, which were particularly wet, would have been lost. It is also hard to imagine how, without them, we would have been able to improve, transform, and make habitable Pixton and its environment in the way we did.

It was also an important time for many of these young people. They found themselves in a community of like-minded people from many different countries between whom many new friendships were born. Many came from Waldorf schools but now met anthroposophy on quite a different level, some later came back to the college as students. It is profoundly important in life to be able, in community with others, to experience giving one's work as a free deed to something that one senses is greater than oneself. Those early summers at Emerson were very special times for those of us involved. There were of course problems, difficulties and upsets, but that is inevitable in a community of free individuals. The fact that many came back in following years, and also recommended the experience to their friends, confirmed the importance of the experience.

The contrast between the summer working holidays and the Christmas experience at the college was a profound polarity. The summer was an outward and widening experience, not only in the outgoing and expansive nature of summer itself, in the nature of the practical work, and the quality of the community, but also in that the young summer workers gave of themselves to something that they experienced as important. In contrast the experience of the 13 holy nights of Christmas as they were celebrated at Emerson was a very inward, quiet, withdrawing, and peaceful time. Many students stayed on over the Christmas period, particularly those who came from distant lands. They could stay either on a working or a paying basis. Many had had no previous experience of such a Christmas, either because they came from non-Christian backgrounds, or because they only experienced the more common form of excessive eating, drinking, and the buying and giving of presents. Many who professed to be Christian spoke of how it was the first time they had really experienced what they felt to be a true Christmas.

The Class 12 Week

In 1972 John Davy initiated the annual Class 12 Week. John was always interested in finding ways to develop and expand the work of the college. He was very aware of the world beyond, and of interesting people and work outside our anthroposophical circles. He saw the importance for the young people at the end of their Waldorf schooling being helped to bridge the gap between their particular education and the wider world into which they would be finding their way. So, with others, he founded the Class 12 Week.

The week was planned in conjunction with the schools. The Emerson summer term ended just before the end of June but the schools' year continued well into July, so the week was planned for early in July to be within the schools' term time, but after Emerson had finished. Costs were kept to a minimum so that all the school-leavers could come. There was no tuition fee. The parents of the Michael Hall Class 12 were asked to house the young people coming from the other schools. Where this was not possible they could camp at the college or certain college rooms could be used as dormitories. The college only charged for meals. All British Waldorf schools with a leaving Class 12 were invited to participate. Not all were able to do so fully, some had different examination commitments. The main ones that fully did so were Edinburgh, Kings Langley, Michael Hall and, more occasionally, Wynstones schools. There were a few years when young people came from schools further afield—from the continent or even the USA. There were usually between 60 and 70 young people who attended.

In Waldorf schools anthroposophy itself is not taught but the education is based on the understanding of the needs of the growing child given by anthroposophy, or spiritual science. Although anthroposophy is not taught, the children become very aware that their education is different from the normal and questions arise. This week was intended to be a time when they could step out of their education into a more adult world where they could be told something about what lay behind their education and have an opportunity to ask questions and be given answers as adults rather than as children still at school. In order to do this in a way in which the children could feel free John felt that their own teachers should not come with them, or if they did, as was necessary for the Edinburgh contingent having to travel overnight, then they would not be allowed into the classes and discussions.

Every year the week was different. John always had some particularly interesting people to come and talk with them; for example, people working practically out of anthroposophy such as a farmer, doctor or banker. He would also invite one or two people from beyond the anthroposophical sphere of activities, people who were active in a particularly interesting, innovative or challenging way. One such memorable occasion was when he invited a group of 'battered wives' and their children supported by Erin Pizzey. (Battered wives was then a term to describe women who suffered regular violence from their husbands.) What a day that was! The children were wild but the Class 12 youngsters were wonderful with them. At the end of the day the visitors almost had to be forced on to the coach, they did not want to leave. It was a very special day for all concerned.

For many it was also important, in meeting others from similar Steiner schools, to find that they were not so different. In meeting these others they came to recognize the value of the education they had had. It could also be a wild week—around 60 young people, suddenly without their teachers and loosed from some of the restraints of childhood. In the early days the smoking was considerable, and if there was nothing on in the evenings they would all disappear down to the pub. But in the discussions and in the questions after lectures they raised profound questions and came to interesting insights. In their freedom they also showed a remarkably serious side.

From those I met in later years I do believe that the week was for many an important event in their stepping into adulthood.

Short Courses and Conferences

I have been able to find only a few prospectuses of the summer activities that developed in the 1970s and '80s. Having researched what records there are I cannot be certain I have always the right dates and details. Life was very full then and somehow we did not get round to keeping diaries, notes or minutes of meetings other than those of the council. Many decisions were actually made in smaller meetings.

Soon after the founding of the Class 12 Week, in around 1973–4, the college began to offer, or host, a number of short summer courses or workshops, at first usually of one week, but later sometimes longer. And in 1980 the college launched into a more regular programme of short courses. These covered a wide variety of subjects but all centred on or arising out of anthroposophy, such as 'Waldorf Education', 'The Spirit of English', 'Discovering the Human Spirit', 'Biodynamic Farming and Gardening', and 'A Music Workshop'. We came to think of these summer courses as a fourth term. We tried to contain them all within a time block of about eight or nine weeks. As these courses increased it became more and more important to have some time when there was nothing happening on the campus in order that there could be a quiet time, a time to breath, and when the necessary cleaning and maintenance could be carried out.

A further development was using the college facilities for hosting larger conferences. One of the first of these was a medical conference in 1978.

The Peace Conferences and Lifeways

In July 1984 John Davy initiated the first of a series of Peace conferences / workshops. The first was titled 'What Makes for Peace?' with Jonathan Porritt, then Co-Chairman of the Ecology Party Council, and Stephanie Leland, founder of the National Council of Women for Life on Earth, as guest speakers. It ran from 13 to 20 July and 84 participants took part. In the mornings there were workshops including 'Conflict and Community Building', 'Peace and the Inner Life', 'In Search of the True Feminine', 'The Healing of Science and Technology', 'Holistic Agriculture', 'Non-Violent Money', and 'The Arts between Tyranny and Chaos'. In the afternoons there were artistic activities including painting, singing, spinning, making poetry, and eurythmy. It was a full and rich programme and very much appreciated by those who took part. The workshops were run by Emerson staff with a number of invited contributors. In the evenings there were lectures or social events. Unfortunately because of the advancing illness that led to his death in October, John was not able to fully participate. He could not give the evening lecture but was very much there in the conference he had initiated. He did give the opening and closing talks.

The following year there was a follow-up conference titled 'Living Peace'. This focused on how to bring peace more actively into our lives and families. It was also highly popular and the number of participants had increased.

During these conferences it had become apparent that many of those attending, if they were to start bringing some of the ideas they met into practice, would need to come with their partners. To make this possible provision would need to be made for them to come as families with arrangements for the children. So out of the Peace conferences 'Lifeways' was born.

In 1986 it was called 'Lifeways Gathering' and advertised as 'The Third International Summer Workshop for Adults and Children at Emerson College'. It included such workshops as 'Birth and Death', 'From Farm to Table' and 'Family-Rhythms and Relationships'. The initiative group for this was Gudrun Davy, Bons Voors, and Linda Churnside. In later years Ann Druitt, who was involved from 1986, and Christine Fynes-Clinton carried the main responsibility for these gatherings, right up to the present, a huge task that has benefited so many people. With few exceptions Lifeways has run every year since it started and is still fulfilling a real need.

These Lifeways gatherings have grown over the years and have been immensely popular, both with the parents and the children. Numbers have had to be limited to below 200, including children. On some occasions over one-third were children. There were crèche arrangements for different age groups for the full mornings. For older children up to 13 there was a camp in the field below Pixton. Various activities were organized for them, including cooking their own meals. These camps were hugely popular. The parents were only allowed minimum contact with their children and so could enjoy the various workshops and activities offered.

★ ★ ★

With all these activities, by the late 1980s there were some years when approaching 1,000 people attended a course, workshop or conference at the college during the summer. A huge problem was providing lodging for them all. In addition to the participants, we had also to provide housing for the young people who kept the place clean and tidy and ready for each course through the summer. We still had only 40 student rooms on campus. Many participants brought tents, but we continued to depend heavily on our landladies. During the peak times for the Lifeways and the big conferences we hired a marquee as an additional dining area. The kitchen was hugely pressed but continued to provide three meals a day seven days a week for all that needed them. We really did not have the facilities to run such a summer programme and provide for so many people. Inevitably many things were inadequate and went wrong, but people continued to come and on the whole spoke very highly of what they met at the college. That itself speaks for their importance.

20
John Davy

After a comparatively short but rapidly developing illness John Davy died on the 28 October 1984 from a tumour in the brain. During the illness he continued to work in the college, though the advancing growth made this more and more difficult for him. It was as though he wished to share with the college community this experience of illness and of the approaching crossing of the threshold with a calm and open acceptance. In this calm acceptance of his approaching death many students came to sense the objective reality of death as a crossing of a threshold, not an end of life. It was indeed like a last gift to them.

For the college community it was a difficult but also a very special time. From our first awareness of the illness it was like a presence in the college, a presence that brought uncertainty—the possibility of having to face great loss and change. It also brought many questions and, perhaps, a challenge to our own convictions—was this really brought about within an all-wise cosmic guidance?

For the rest I do not think I can do better than leave it to extracts from articles Francis Edmunds and John Thomson wrote in the 1985 New Year Letter to Friends, and part of a letter Gudrun Davy wrote.

Extract from Francis Edmunds:

> *Dear Emersonians and Friends of Emerson College,*
> *And thus it was that he gave up a highly successful career to join Emerson College, at first half-time, and later full-time. I have been praised for my good judgement in appointing him. It was not quite like that really. He came inevitably, as with the other events in his life, when the time for it was right. He once said to me, rather wonderingly, that he had never seemed to have the trials and struggles in life that others had. His life did indeed move from phase to phase with ease and certainty as by a special grace.*
>
> *By degrees John came to take over the major responsibility for the Foundation Year on which the rest of the life of the college is based. It was a work which he dearly loved. It fell to him to make the connection in writing and in person with all the incoming students for that year, men and women mainly in their 20s and 30s, from 20 countries and more, with their different backgrounds, trainings, and professions, and all in search of values giving*

meaning to life. It was now for John, assisted by his colleagues to get to know the students individually, help them, advise them, guide them on their way to discovering their further goals in life. The students learnt to appreciate him deeply for his knowledge and clarity of exposition, his live interest in contemporary theory and research, his inner freedom and openness of mind, his care and warmth of understanding for each one, and beyond that, his wide interest in the human endeavours of others—for all this they esteemed and loved him.

Helen Glover, in an epistle of some length, reviews what her two years at Emerson College have meant to her. Towards the end she refers to 'the Peace Week which, though outside the Emerson Year, was one of the most important things for me, because I identified with it completely, somehow. It was exactly what I had hoped would happen, but of course, it was John Davy's brilliant instinct and determination that began it all. I have never learnt so much about how a new idea is realized in a community, as I learnt at the staff meeting I was privileged to attend . . . This magical beginning was also the impetus that perhaps carried everyone even when John fell ill.'

Helen ends her review: 'On a personal level, if one's adult life in the world can be said to have a godfather, then John Davy has been mine; he has not only respected what I am but encouraged it, which has seemed to me like receiving from him the gift of freedom, or key of gold.'

The words which follow are from a letter from Rainbow Rosenbloom whom many will remember. He is at present class teacher to the 5th Grade of the Waldorf School in Santa Cruz. He writes, having heard of John's death:

'John was very special to me—different from anyone else in the movement. I experienced a man of integrity and deep commitment, yet one who knew how to embrace a fellow sans judgement. He wasn't afraid of showing emotion he felt; his honesty was always apparent. His connection with work in the world was a priority in his life; again, in the spirit of embracing as opposed to alienating. He was so unpretentious as a spiritual seeker, penetrating, yet first and foremost a man of the earth. I always remember the work days at Emerson—John was there with the rest of us dealing with muck—always smiling. That is the picture I have of him as I write—forever smiling as he works.'

I cannot now list the many innovations John introduced, not only into the Foundation Year but into the work of the college as a whole—always in the direction of better communication and more inward co-operation, and always in readiness to appreciate and give support to initiatives as these arose in others. It is amazing how, in the last weeks of his life he would awaken morning after morning with a new thought or image for the progress of the college, not as an institution for itself, but rather as a place where things could be practised and values tested which might then contribute more widely to life. For example, he called urgently for finding the being, Natura, once again; we live alongside her but not with her and in her. He offered practical suggestions whereby Natura might, in daily life and work, once again become alive for us. Indeed he left behind him a sheaf of thoughts of one kind and another. Sifting them out and studying them now, makes him very present.

Illness always conceals a mystery—why that particular illness for that particular person at that given moment in life—and every illness entails to some degree, a battle with death. Of all illnesses, none can be more invidious than cancer. It creeps in like a thief in the night into whatever part of the organism it will, at any age, takes silent hold, and when finally discovered, is generally too late. So it was with John. He appeared to be still in the flood of life, spiritually and also physically, with far-seeing vision for new works, enterprises, for the future; then symptoms set in, signs of physical debility and the diagnosis was an advanced condition of a tumour in the brain. It was as though a dark evil fell across his path where he was striving most ardently for light. At a moment when the danger seemed most imminent the college was assembled and it was asked that we think of John not as though lying prostrate, but as erect in spirit and fearless, which indeed he was all through. He made his body, even with its growing disabilities, subservient to his will as long as was possible. The thought of an operation had to be set aside. Other treatments were resorted to but proved ultimately to be of no avail. John continued to work. He even began the term taking a group of students for The Philosophy of Freedom *as he had done in previous years. He actually met his group, though with difficulty and with Gudrun by, on the Monday of his last week. He died on the Sunday following, the 28th of October. The body had to succumb.*

Gudrun tells how determined John was to visit Tintagel again, to meet the King of the Elements, as he put it. Twice he climbed that steep promontory with the ancient seat of the Court of King Arthur down below, this despite disabilities already setting in. It confirmed the image one could hardly fail to have that hidden behind the illness was a knight in armour fighting evil. Rudolf Steiner, after visiting Tintagel, had spoken wonderful words about the Arthurian Fellowship whose origin he dated back to several centuries before Christ's descent to earth. He spoke of the knights, quoting St Augustine, as pre-Christian Christians and described them as being under the guidance of the Archangel Michael, and of Christ as the Sun-Spirit reigning in the

Cosmos—hence the expression King of the Elements. He had spoken also of the meeting of the Grail Stream coming from the East with the Arthurian Stream of the West; of Christ, after His incarnation, advancing from the East to meet His own Image in the West. With all this John was fully familiar and felt deeply connected. Rudolf Steiner had also spoken of Chartres, which John loved and where he had lectured, as the meeting place of the Arthurian and Grail mysteries in the teachings of the great Masters who had founded it. We can imagine how vividly and powerfully these images must have lived in John, with his body already beginning to fail him, as he stood on that great rock in the West, looking across towards America of the New World which he had also come to know, with the surging waves on either side and the ancient site of Arthur below.

On September 28th he woke with a message for Michaelmas Day, the 29th. He and Gudrun were there for the College Festival in the morning which included some eurythmy, Julian Pook's Michaelmas Song, and the Michaelmas address, shared, as had become customary, by a student and a member of staff. It was arranged for John to give a talk in the evening. The Foundation Studio was packed every inch. He spoke of many symptoms and tendencies of the present time in a strongly Michaelmas mood stressing where there was hope, nor was humour lacking. He received an ovation of prolonged heart-felt clapping. It was a triumphant moment. He remained upright and fearless as from the beginning. His spirit prevailed until close to the end when his physical body could no longer hold out and had to succumb.

To me, as I write this now, and as I dared to pronounce in the funeral address, it has seemed plain that behind John's illness there lived a great resolve. It lay in the pattern of his life, moving from phase to phase as each presented itself.

Where, we ask, is humanity to find the moral powers to meet and curb and overcome the gathering forces of evil, of disruption and destruction we see stretching through all the world, where but through deeds of sacrifice? Perhaps we may be permitted to see that even as John left a highly successful career to devote himself to an anthroposophical task that needed him, so, having brought his gifts and capabilities to a peak point in regards to his given life-time, having thus reached a new phase, he crossed the border, for a further stage of fulfilment, into the spiritual world, that what he had acquired thus far might be transmuted and enhanced to levels of a heightened morality with which to meet, in a further life, the dire needs of humanity on earth.

I sent John a note from America, too late to reach him, but perhaps not the thought it embodied. It contained the following words. 'I felt from the first that you are fighting a great battle for us all, and this conviction grows with me. Whatever the gods may decree, whatever their reasons, I know in my heart that you cannot fail.'

This does not diminish the tragedy. We feel most deeply with Gudrun whose heroism in this ordeal we all here have witnessed, and with their three sons and daughter, and with Charles Davy, John's father, also with Richard, John's brother, and his family. We feel horribly the absence of John's presence in our midst and in so many different places. And yet we know that John in the spirit would not wish us to shed tears for him, but rather that we follow his gaze where he now is, with forward looking front.

Extract from John Thomson (also from the 1985 New Year Letter to Friends):

The reports on past work, the projects for new work which these pages will try to bring to you at this New Year time must all carry a deep sense of the loss which the staff and students have experienced in the death of our dear friend and colleague, John Davy. Right until the end, John did not withdraw in thought or deed from the warmest concern for the future of Emerson College. From the time that his illness declared itself, we were the witnesses of his daily preoccupations with the well-being of our work. Regularly, in the summer months, letters and draft proposals containing ideas and guidelines for the development of the College work were delivered by John or by Gudrun into the hands of various staff members for our consideration and discussion 'if wanted'.

What became known as John Davy's document which reassembled and developed further the content of the various letters was completed by John at the end of August. John was still able to be with us in some of the meetings of the General Faculty in late September and early October. The Faculty wished to make the document the basis of extensive discussion on the aims and tasks of the College. John shared these first discussions. Of course some of the ideas, something of the perspective which he had set down for us, was not unfamiliar. But this intensive search for a fresh cohesion in our work, the strong impulse towards a renewal of the vision, this energetic drive to find a purposeful integration of aims, work and community—these were John's. John bequeathed to us a new dedication. We carry from the year in which we mourned his departure into this 1985, a strength, a faith and a hope, which he had helped us to understand, in the work that Emerson College was founded to serve.

It will not be out of place here if I give something (it can be no more than a suggestion) of the questions that most concern us and to which we must make our response in the times that lie immediately ahead. It will be most suitable, if I refer to John's document in which many of these questions were clearly posed.

As the work at Emerson has evolved over 21 years, there has been a continual reaffirmation of Francis Edmunds's original vision and founding impulse. In last year's report, John Davy gave in characteristic style, a broad ranging and thorough survey of the achievements of the College and how it stood in the world on reaching maturity. He wrote 'The future will undoubtedly be full of surprises and extremely challenging. But the authenticity of what was begun 21 years ago and the potential for the future are unmistakable'.

To justify this confidence, this sense of the validity of the undertaking, a spirit of enquiry, of questioning, a readiness to probe and reassess our practice must always be present. In the document referred to, John Davy invited his colleagues to an investigation of problems that emerge from our work. Such a venture obliges us to move from seeing certain features of college life and study as simply part of the nature of things to seeing them as symptoms of our inner and outer habits. Overloading, stress and digestion (psychic rather than gastric) are recognized only too often as inmates in our anthroposophical training centres. There is often too much concentration on the richness of the ingredients of curriculum in such places. This emphasis on variety of content can be seen as an opponent to another element which Steiner pointed to as an objective in the Waldorf school approach: economy. To understand what is meant by economy, we have to proceed in a direction other than the one leading to content. We must look at method, rhythm, the process of learning, the practice, the intimate and mysterious relationship between knowing and doing.

Emerson was built on its Foundation Year. Now some nine second-year training courses surround it. These training courses have not only to understand their aims and search out right methods but to grapple with the question 'What is a sound foundation for our work?'. This requires an examination of the relationship between Foundation Year and Training Courses. This process was begun in the course of last year. The new step prompted by John's document is to understand more thoroughly the whole process from the student's initial encounter with anthroposophy to his or her work as a trained professional. John Davy envisaged this process in three stages:

Foundation Work
Basic Training
Professionalisation

These stages were not seen as arbitrary but as belonging to an archetypal process. John drew his suggestion in part from the 'Young Doctors' lectures, (especially the lecture of 8/11/24) in which Steiner outlines three fundamental steps in the training of doctors. First course: a foundation in the study of man and nature. Second course: an 'esoteric deepening' into the 'medical forces'. Final course: awakening the moral capacities, notably the courage and will to heal. Such an outline is perhaps indicative also of the training steps required by the student teacher, student farmer, etc.

It is not possible to pursue this enquiry further here. It is however, important for us to indicate to you something of this legacy which John Davy left us—a legacy that typifies the man. 'Here are thoughts, suggestions, themes for investigation. Some light and encouragement for the way forward', he seems to say. 'Can we not work on these together?' We can have perhaps a deep awareness that we are indeed working on these together . . .

An extract from a letter Gudrun Davy sent to all those who had written to her:

During his illness John became more and more aware that we have to constantly rethink our life situation and keep it in movement and development. He felt that Emerson College was a place where people could find help with this process and from which help would flow out to contribute towards healing the ills of our time. Summer conferences like the one on 'What makes for Peace?' and several others brought more and more people to Emerson to exchange ideas, to find a measure of harmony, and to leave enriched. This gave John a deep satisfaction but also an urgent feeling that more could be done in this direction.

In the last few weeks John spoke to me often of his love for Emerson College and of his vision for an ever greater potential to reach out further into the world. On a practical level, however, that would mean improvements and enlargements to the buildings. He said that perhaps this year the beginnings of improvements for the kitchen/dining room area could be thought of, as the architectural plans already existed. This would make it more possible to have larger conferences and would help those who prepare the food with the special care that we all have grown accustomed to at the College.

As some people have already sent money instead of flowers I thought it fitting to describe John's great wish to you with the hope that one or the other person might still contribute to this 'John Davy Memorial Fund', which has come into being of its own accord.

21
Francis Edmunds—His Task Completed

Francis Edmunds spoke at the funeral of John Davy, the man he had planned and thought would continue the work he had founded. It was indeed a poignant moment. Francis himself was now 82 years old. He was as though uncertain whether he should step back into some sort of leadership. In his time he had been the single founder and leader. John had moved the leadership from the single individual to the group of colleagues working together. Though John had gone, there was still an active leadership of good people. Francis had an invitation to attend the Council of Management meetings whenever he wished but had seldom done so recently and was very out of touch with the day-to-day matters in the life of the college. But he did, nevertheless, carry within himself a concern as to the future leadership of the college.

Francis continued, where wanted, to work with students through occasional lectures, study groups and through personal conversations. Many valued what he still had to give, and benefited enormously, but increasingly into the late 1980s he had less and less connection with and understanding of the generation then coming as students to the college. As I described earlier, Emerson College was founded for the young seekers of a particular generation, those who came into their adulthood in the 1960s and '70s. He told me once that he sometimes had the feeling that he was of their generation but had come early in order to prepare a place for them. But now, in the mid-1980s the students were already of a later and different generation. They were not on quite the same search, they had different questions. In the earlier days the students had flocked to his lectures—which were deeply valued and inspiring. But now, though many still valued and received much from them, there were an increasing number who got little from him; some of whom would even say, for example, 'What is the old man talking about, I cannot understand what he says?' He no longer had that immediate connection with these young people.

Francis had always had a love and understanding for Shakespeare. Connected to this was his sense of the importance of the English language as a world language. He saw clearly what was perhaps not so obvious as it is today, that if anthroposophy was to reach out to the world, as it was intended to do, then for many people it would only be accessible through the English language. But he experienced that this was not understood in the German-speaking anthroposophical circles. In the early days he and his impulse for Emerson College had been recognized and had received active support in America, but to a much less extent in Europe and in England. When, towards the end of his life he took this question up with the Vorstand in Dornach he came away feeling that he was still not understood.

These were not easy times for him.

In 1987, Elliot Hiller, a eurythmist who had visited Emerson and given lectures on drugs, spoke to Francis of Gideon Fontalba, founder of the School of the White Source, whom it was suggested was an initiate. From his early searches Francis had always hoped to meet an initiate. Francis had arranged to visit the Vorstand in Dornach. It was arranged that after this visit Elliot Hiller would take Francis to meet Fontalba, which he did. John Meeks and Carol Fraser, who had met Fontalba before, were also present. At the meeting Francis invited Fontalba to visit Emerson College. During the visit of Fontalba to Emerson a number of meetings were arranged; some for small groups but some also for all members of the college

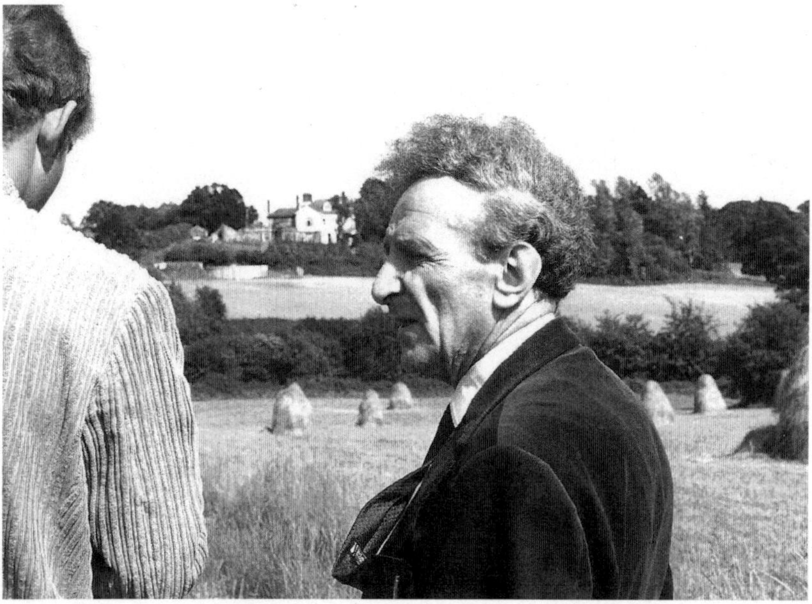

Francis Edmunds, with Pixton in the background

including a number of specially invited anthroposophists from London and the local area.

It is not my intention to describe or comment on these meetings, but to say that while Francis and a few colleagues had confidence that Gideon Fontabla was what he claimed to be, the great majority of the staff of the college as well as older and experienced anthroposophists who met him were equally certain that he was not, but that he was trying to insinuate himself into, or even take over, the college. If Francis himself had not been involved, this might have been dealt with without too much difficulty. But as it was it was clearly a serious situation that had to be faced and dealt with. The whole future of the college was seen to be at stake.

John Thomson played an essential and leading role in helping guide the college through to as satisfactory a resolution as it was probably possible to reach. There were many discussions in meetings of the whole staff, the Faculty, the Council of Management, and with the individual people concerned. There were certain guiding principles established or understood for resolving this issue: it was a matter for the college itself to resolve without involvement of anyone from outside; the process should be as open, fair and transparent as possible and include all members of staff who should then be ready to stand behind the decision; where necessary the student body should also be involved; and it must be dealt with on the highest and most human level possible without recourse to legal process.

After many discussions John and Doris Meeks and Carol Fraser accepted that they could not be allowed to continue working in the college while they continued in any way to be involved with, or influenced by, Gideon Fontalba. The college would continue to pay their salaries for some months to give them time to sort out their future.

For Francis it was very difficult. No one suggested that he should leave. He himself admitted that he found himself caught in between—sitting on the fence as he termed it. There was, of course, no question of his commitment to anthroposophy as given by Rudolf Steiner. The question was whether Gideon Fontalba also worked on the basis of those same spiritual truths, or whether what he taught was some sort of distortion of it. Francis accepted the decisions arrived at by the college while he felt the uncertainty of himself not being able to decide, as he put it, on which side of the fence to come down. He continued at the college but tended to withdraw more into himself.

By the late 1980s most of those for whom the college was originally created had been and were now out in the world in the full flow of their work—though there would continue to be others who carried the same questions, they were an ever-decreasing group. The world was changing and the later generations of young people brought with them new and different impulses, questions and needs. The numbers in the Foundation Year had already started to reduce in 1981–2—it was the training courses that continued to flourish. John Davy who had taken on the leadership of the Foundation Year had died in 1984, but Francis lived on, seemingly without a role, writing his book—posthumously published as *Quest for Meaning**—and continued, when needed, to lecture.

Was there truly a diminishing role for a Foundation Year Course? Were there not other young people who had brought with them into the world resolves on future work but who now needed somewhere like Emerson College to help them on to their destiny paths? The world had changed; humanity itself was evolving as the consciousness soul continued to awaken in a rapidly expanding number of human souls around the world. However important and good the training courses were it is hard to believe that a new form of Foundation Year was not needed still, that there were not many young people in the world looking for just such a place, but one formed not only around the questions and needs of their later time, but also where they would find in the very structure and social fabric of the college a living expression of the spiritual needs of the time and of the near future.

★ ★ ★

Up to 1989, when Francis died, a little under 1,800 students had been through the Foundation Year. Others came directly into the training courses and many more into the short courses. The story of Emerson is really the sum of all the individual stories of these, mostly young, people—how they came and what they gained at the college and how they took something of this out into the world, into their work, into their schools, farms and other communities and into their families. The work Francis started was now out in the world—there it continues.

★ ★ ★

In the later part of the 1980s it seemed his work was done. On Monday 13 November 1989, just after speaking at the College Meeting about death and the importance of working with the dead, he himself passed peacefully across the threshold into the Spiritual World.

---

* Francis Edmunds, *Quest for Meaning* (London: Bloomsbury, 1998).

With Roswitha, I was at that time in America. Just then we were visiting Christopher and Martina Mann in Wisconsin. Herbert Koepf and Georg Locher were also there when the message came through that Francis had died. Roswitha, Georg, and Christopher immediately returned to Forest Row. I had a commitment to give four lectures at the Waldorf Schools Economic Conference in Fair Oaks so it was thought better that I do that and then return. So, as I was not present for the few days after Francis's death, I think it best that I include here extracts from articles written by Paul Matthews and by Georg Locher, his son-in-law, published in the 1990 edition of the Emerson College Newsletter *Circles*:

Paul Matthews—editorial in *Circles* 1990

Francis Edmunds was a man who trusted he had the right to exist. In the way he walked from his house to his work at the College, or back home afterwards, there was not a shadow of doubt. He was forever stepping with courage into the next moment of himself, and to see this gave others confidence for their own existence. Even the manner of his death had that same decisiveness. He had spoken at the College House-meeting about Remembrance Sunday and the need to establish a creative relationship with the dead. And then half an hour later while having supper at home he simply died. He died simply. His deeds were words, and his words deeds, firing those who heard with a sense of urgency for their tasks. Often at College staff meetings he would listen intently for a while, and then his foot would start tapping and you knew that a word was working its way up, very often with the intent of placing the work of the College within a larger spiritual context. During his last days he stood up in the College dining-room waving his newspaper to make sure that we were sufficiently awake to the events in Eastern Europe—'a great in-pouring of light' as he expressed it.

This linking of the destiny of the College with wider events was absolutely apparent during his last moments. Having spoken so movingly about the Dead (including those killed during the two world wars) he sat down, and Tadeu Caldas of the Rural Development Programme began to speak about his witness of events in Berlin as the Wall was being opened. And at the end of his talk he presented Francis with a piece from the Wall—it was received with a great smile of satisfaction.

Looking back now on that moment in the light of subsequent events it seems somehow to be the signature of all that Francis worked for. Twenty-eight years earlier, realising that young people were being served stones for bread, he had 'set up a school for adults in which the true image of Man may be recognised so that from it may flow the inspiration to permeate earthly knowledge with cosmic wisdom, and human action with individual morality'—these are the words from his first Prospectus of Emerson College. So, when the turbulent year of 1968 arrived, and the walls of conventional education could not contain the energies of the rising generation, the College was ready to receive them. The period that followed was the heyday of Francis's work, and certainly there must be thousands of people across the globe who feel immensely grateful to him for having founded a place where their ideals could be recognised and their creative energies directed.

Twenty-one years have passed since that earlier 'in-pouring of the light', and though in Eastern Europe at that time those energies were blocked, the ideal of the free human being that people on both sides of the Wall continued to carry, and the growing awareness of our responsibility for the one Earth, could not be contained forever within the imposed boundaries; and we are seeing the consequences. It is my strong hope that Francis can see his work now in the context of these large events, and I would like to say to him: When you received the meaning of that piece of stone in your hand the moment became transparent, a moment for the true Being and significance of this College that you founded. And when you then passed it around for all those present to share (and there are 30 nations here this year) it became bread in our hands through a grace which even you could not have expected in your lifetime . . .

A Tribute to Francis Edmunds
Georg Locher

Three Kings' Day, and I am flying West again to visit and help in many schools; flying too under the star of Waldorf education which had shone with such force in the destiny of Francis. How many hours of his life he must have spent on board ship, or later mainly on board airship, on or above the Atlantic, reflecting, preparing, communing with the impulse he was serving. For decades he worked untiringly in education on both sides of this historic ocean with the Southern Hemisphere, South Africa, Australia and New Zealand, also receiving him frequently for inspiration and awakening calls.

I had just completed a week in the Toronto Waldorf School, which had culminated in a teacher-development conference with 40 teachers from the five Ontario Waldorf Schools, when, arriving in the Mid West, the news of Francis's sudden death on Monday, 13th November, 1989 reached me. The news spread like wildfire around the world. During the following days and weeks, he must have lived strongly in the hearts of those who knew him and who met together in many memorial gatherings throughout the world he had travelled. Cutting my trip short and having arrived back for the large College memorial meeting, he seemed to be present in extra strength though having left the physical plane behind. His still youthful expression, the many friends and messages from near and far, the flowers, wreaths and shared memories: The College was celebrating its founder by experiencing the loss of this powerful individuality who had carried the anthroposophical cause into the hearts of so many.

Preparing for the funeral address which was to include basic biographical aspects of his rich life, I was struck again by the fact that his crowning life's work, the founding and directing of Emerson College, had grown out of his teaching and pioneering involvement in Waldorf Education:

Francis, the class teacher, Francis, the teacher of adolescents and developer of Upper or High Schools, Francis the teacher trainer and adult educator, Francis, the teacher of teachers, the lecturer and inspirer, the travelling ambassador for Steiner's renewal of childhood education so urgently needed in the apocalyptic unfolding of our 5th Post-Atlantean Epoch.

I met Francis first when I was 16 years old, joining Michael Hall School as a foreign student. He taught us science and religion. He was a fulfilling educational experience, strong and direct, never mind the subject or whether the scientific experiments worked or not. His full and loud laughter (often on the in-breath), as he sat casually on a desk in the religion lessons, telling us about Socrates, will continue to ring in my ears. He was always down to earth, yet non-pedestrian, intuitive and creative in his clear articulated thinking, filling the classroom with his mighty ego and always giving one an inner lift and sometimes a push and a pull in one's sleepy will region whilst remaining totally objective and leaving one free.

This I also experienced when Francis, seven years later, became my teacher in the Michael Hall Teachers' Training Course. There was a strong sense of mission in Francis which sparked over to his students. The present moment was always laced with a sense of future and life had no ceiling—in his presence! For me too, as I know from many others, Francis was the gateway to my conscious anthroposophy.

I loved his English, which for my Swiss ears, was rather un-English in its clear, full and very expressive articulation. Only later did I discover that Francis only arrived in England at the age of seven and with his Jewish-Russian background was indeed one of those 'homeless' souls pre-destined to

> *the awakening of the consciousness soul, making the English language his 'conscious own' in a deeply cosmopolitan way.*
>
> *As a teacher trainer and adult educator, his main course contribution was always his creative Study of Man, based on Steiner's 14 lectures given to the first group of teachers in 1919. He re-created and created. There was no easy taking notes or recording contents for future reference. The lessons were received as awakening will impulses, as powerful calls for moral and vocational commitment.*
>
> *Religion, Science and Art all flowed together in Francis's lessons, lectures and addresses. He was a specialist at being a generalist, integrating the phenomena of life with the realities of the spirit, the proof of which was Francis himself in action and what went on between him and his participants, beyond words and meanings. Above all he was able to communicate trust, trust in one's own resources and potentials, and trust in evolution and our times which call for active doing . . .*

And at his funeral address (part of which I have included in chapter 2) Georg ended with the words:

> *Francis was a person foremost of will and intuition. He mastered the fiery choleric temperament and impatience of his younger years and became a deeply compassionate listener and counsellor, as well as remaining the youthful, uplifting speaker who, often with down-to-earth humour, made the spirit a creative experience of the moment, right up to his last day. The future was always with him and around him. Living longer than his chosen successor as principal of the College, John Davy, he was always looking and searching, really beyond the end of this century, for the succession to the work he had started.*
>
> *As the truly moral and Christian force he is, he will surely continue to pioneer the education needed in this epoch of evolution, albeit now on the other side. Here he will live on in the striving, teaching and work of his students and colleagues. We feel deepest gratitude and a sense of great privilege to have met and worked with Francis Edmunds.*

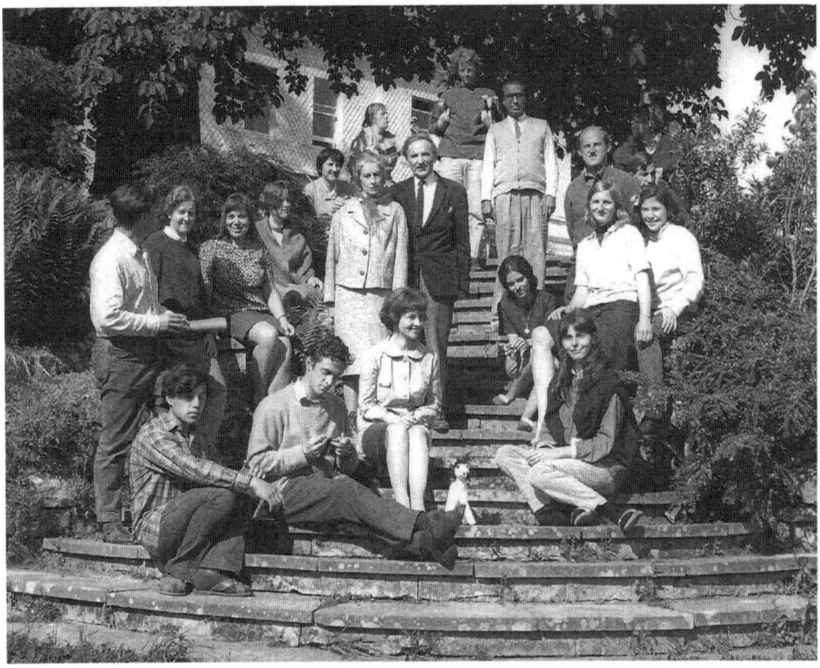

Students with Francis and Elizabeth Edmunds standing in the centre

22
Final Thoughts

Inevitably the question thrusts itself forward; why was it not possible for Emerson College to continue, why did it go into decline? If it was such an important place for so many in the 1960s, '70s and '80s did it really have to come to an end? Surely there were others of the following generations who needed something like the Foundation Year.

I could not, and do not intend to try, to give any sort of full answer to these questions. Looking back over the years there are many causes that could be given as reasons for this gradual reversal of its earlier growth, both from within the college and from events and changes in the world at large. Here I would like to point to just a few of what I think were important factors that came from within the college itself. The main ones that have often been cited and certainly had their effects, for example the burden of increased health and safety legislation, the clamping down on visas for students from beyond Europe, and the need for accreditation of the courses, all came well after the reduction in numbers had begun.

As I explained earlier, Francis founded the college to meet the questions and needs of the young people of a particular time; the 1960s and beyond. John Davy and others joined him in that work. There is much that points to the fact that the work as originally founded was completed by the end of the 1980s. I indicated some evidence of this earlier: student numbers in the Foundation Year began falling off around 1982, that is, before, not after, John died; Francis himself had a very different relationship to the students of the later time; John had already hinted at finding new tasks—his illness and death could also be seen as pointing to this.

After 1982 the training courses continued to grow for a time, and then their numbers also began dropping off. These, particularly the smaller courses, had been able to continue as they did so long as there was a substantial Foundation Year. It was the Foundation Year that covered the main financial overheads of the college, and also attracted students who then went on into the training courses. The college as a whole also depended on the continuation of the Foundation Year for the 'ethos' that had given the college a worldwide reputation and attracted so many people to it.

The training courses could be viable within the whole while that whole included a Foundation Year which was over half the whole. In this situation the training courses developed what seemed a comfortable way of working—with low student numbers and a relatively high ratio of staff to students. But as the Foundation Year reduced in numbers the training courses could not pick up the increased share of the overheads without considerably increasing the fees needed to keep them going.

There we come to what for me was the real question: why were students not now finding their way to Emerson? Again, many different reasons could be given for this. The need to go more immediately into work and the need for recognized qualifications have often been cited. But these were problems from the beginning. They may have grown, but I do believe that if there had really been the will in more young people to come, as there had been earlier, they would have found ways. Another factor was that other similar colleges and training courses had come into being. But none of these had the same quality of all embracing international and social/cultural life that was maintained at Emerson.

There is no doubt in my mind that as the older people who carried the anthroposophical base of the college moved on, retired or died, particularly following the deaths of John Davy and then Francis Edmunds, the anthroposophical foundations on which the college was founded were slowly but progressively lost sight of. It seemed that there were not the people to continue the leadership of the college on the deeper anthroposophical foundations on which it had been founded and continued to be formed during its earlier years of growth. I was not directly involved in the teaching, but my sense was that while anthroposophy continued to live in the actual course work in the Foundation Year and most of, but not all the training courses, over time it gradually disappeared from the practice in much of the rest of the college. It disappeared from the administrative structure and its procedures and also from many parts of the social life, including the Festivals. This resulted in a certain dishonesty entering into the life and spiritual environment of the college.

I will give two examples out of many possible ones.

As I mentioned in chapter 2 in relationship to Adam Bittleston, anthroposophical spiritual science points to the Christ event and the Mystery of Golgotha as objective historical and spiritual facts which played an essential and pivotal role in human evolution. An understanding of this need not depend on, and can be quite separate from, any particular religious beliefs or teaching. Knowledge of this was an important aspect of the college at its founding. The main Christian Festivals were celebrated at the college out of this understanding—they were not primarily religious events.

But there came a time during the 1990s when increasingly there was a reluctance to mention the word Christ, or Christian, particularly in regard to the Festivals. We always had a number of students from other religious cultures and there was a feeling that we should not discriminate between the different faiths. This was reinforced by the fact that many of those students who did come from a Christian background had for one reason or another lost faith in it. The reluctance to speak of Christ because of the word's religious connotations meant that the Festivals themselves began slowly to lose much of their original spiritual substance and meaning.

This seemed to indicate that there were no longer the teachers at the college who could reach beyond the particular needs of their courses and bring an understanding of the anthroposophical perception of the nature of the Christ Being, of his mission, and its relevance for all humanity to the diverse group of students that came to the college. It seemed also to indicate that the reality of the role of destiny and karma as an essential factor behind students finding their way to the college had been lost sight of. It was always possible that some of these students had been led by their destiny to Emerson just in order to find their way to the Christ as an objective fact rather than as a Christian teaching.

The second example is that there came a time in, if I remember rightly, the early '90s when the word 'marketing' came increasingly to replace the word 'publicity' or 'advertising'. To make an issue of this might seem as being rather pedantic over something of minor importance, but it was an indication of the start of a trend of deep significance for the college.

Within the college there had always been the knowledge that the people for whom the college was created would not come just because, for example, they saw an advertisement, or needed certain qualifications. A person's destiny, which carries also his pre-birth intentions, works through the will, not through thinking. As I have pointed to earlier, Francis often said to a student 'It is your feet that brought you here, not your head.'

Certainly publicity is often needed. If a person decides to go to a particular place he may need to find a signpost that points the way. But it is not the signpost that persuades him to go to there. The intention to find such a place had already been made elsewhere and at a different time. When those working in such an institution as Emerson start using the word 'marketing' it is a clear indication that they have lost sight of the objective reality of destiny and karma and also of the original spiritual foundations of the college. They might still talk about destiny and karma and of the spiritual world in the classrooms, but they act out of a quite different knowledge. They now speak and act out of that which is true for the economic sphere of human activity but that can only work destructively when applied to the cultural spiritual life.

In other ways too, the direction from which the college found its inner life and form began to change. As I have already indicated, Francis Edmunds was in many ways ahead of his time. From the beginning the college was informed, not only in its purpose and spiritual task but also in its practical organization, its administrative and financial arrangements, and its legal structure, out of the future. That is, its structure and practices were formed out of an intuitive understanding of that towards which humanity was evolving—the further awakening of the consciousness soul. But increasingly more conventional ways of thinking and old established administrative procedures and structures, ones that had their roots in the old hierarchical and theocratic societies of the past, began to take over. These were often referred to as being more professional.

When in an anthroposophical organization the people leading it are able to take the anthroposophy right into the practical life, into the administration, structure, and daily working—when the organization as a social being in all its aspects becomes a living expression of anthroposophy in practice, then that organization will be seen to be formed out of its own inherent threefold nature. The threefold social order is there, even if it is not planned or applied. Of course it greatly strengthens the organization if one can, through an actual study of the threefold nature of human social life, work consciously on that which begins to arise anyway, only unconsciously.

When such an organization as Emerson College is enabled to form itself in accordance with the inherent threefold nature of human society, of which it is a part, then the people who come to it will feel akin to it, will feel in their souls free and at home within it as an outer form reflecting their own threefold nature.

Emerson College reached a nadir in its life towards the end of 2009. Student numbers had continued to decline, particularly for the Foundation Year and Education Courses. It seemed that what was now being offered by the college was not what was being looked for by sufficient numbers of people of this later time. Their questions were different from the questions of 30 years earlier and there were not the people in the college able to find a new task in the greatly changed conditions of the world in order to meet the individual and social challenges faced by the new generations.

As a consequence of the resulting serious financial shortfall, in February 2010 the decision was taken by the then trustees, on advice from financial consultants, to close the college. On Saturday 27 March 2010 there was a final closing ceremony to which many friends came.

But, independently, three people had already come forward determined to find a way to save the college—Fumiko Chikami, Dr John Lees, and, separately, Robert Lord. They decided to work together and put forward proposals which were accepted by the creditors, trustees, and consultant accountants. They were appointed as the new trustees in April 2010.

Something new is now slowly trying to arise on the old Emerson campus. They have to find a new task and future for the college, something that will also continue the 'special place' quality that is still experienced by some people coming onto the Pixton campus. They are determined that what does emerge will be firmly grounded in anthroposophy.

★ ★ ★

For many years now, ever since the 1990s when it was clear that our numbers were steadily declining, I have carried the question: are there not now also young people looking for a place where they will find help on to their path of inner development and spiritual work as there was in the 1960s, '70s and into the '80s, and for whom Francis founded Emerson College? If there are such people, and I have no doubt there are many, what are their questions now, what do they need to help them as then they were helped by the Foundation Year?

To where do they go to prepare themselves for their work in the world? And will it need to be so very different as some people have suggested?